D1323093

"*Counterclockwise* presents a new way to think about lifelong health and aging. Read this most important book to improve your quality of life at any age."
—DEEPAK CHOPRA, M.D.

"*Counterclockwise* is a gem—a book that is equally practical and philosophical without seeming to be either, and one that makes you feel better—more conscious and more prepared—about growing old, even if you weren't feeling bad about it in the first place. There is no one thinking more creatively about sickness and health than Ellen Langer, and she shares what she knows here with uncommon felicity."
—SUE HALPERN, author of *Can't Remember What I Forgot: The Good News from the Frontlines of Memory Research*

"Take a brilliant, creative social scientist, without any respect for conventional wisdom and you get Ellen Langer. She is a fantastic storyteller, and *Counterclockwise* is a fascinating story about the unexpected ways in which our minds and bodies are connected. More important, *Counterclockwise* shows how a better understanding of this relationship can lead to a better life."
—DAN ARIELY, PH.D., author of *Predictably Irrational: The Hidden Forces That Shape Our Decisions*

"Ellen Langer's work has been an inspiration to me for years. *Counterclockwise,* her latest book, will change the way you think about your health—for the better. It's simply fabulous."
—CHRISTIANE NORTHRUP, M.D., author of *The Wisdom of Menopause* and *The Secret Pleasures of Menopause*

"Ellen Langer has used her extensive research and scholarship to write a book that will be indispensable to anyone confronting illness or old age (in other words, to everyone). She shows that many seemingly unavoidable damages to our body can be reversed or ameliorated by the conscious application of the mind. The book can be used as a manual against despair, but more than that, it is a seminal work in what the author calls 'the psychology of possibility'—a perspective on the unexplored riches of human nature."

—MIHALY CSIKSZENTMIHALYI, PH.D., author of *Flow: The Psychology of Optimal Experience*

About the Author

Ellen J. Langer was the first woman to be tenured in psychology at Harvard where she is still Professor of Psychology, and a member of the Division on Aging of the Faculty of Medicine. Dr Langer is the author of eleven books and over two hundred research articles. She lives in Cambridge, M.A.

Also By

Mindfulness
The Power of Mindful Learning
On Becoming an Artist

COUNTER CLOCKWISE

COUNTER CLOCKWISE

ELLEN J. LANGER

A Proven Way to Think Yourself Younger and Healthier

HODDER

First published in Great Britain in 2010 by Hodder & Stoughton
An Hachette UK company

First published in paperback in 2010

1

A CIP catalogue record for this title is available from the British Library

ISBN 978 0 340 99476 4

Printed and bound by CPI Mackays, Chatham ME5 8TD

Hodder & Stoughton policy is to use papers that are natural, renewable
and recyclable products and made from wood grown in sustainable forests.
The logging and manufacturing processes are expected to conform to the
environmental regulations of the country of origin.

Hodder & Stoughton Ltd
338 Euston Road
London NW1 3BH

www.hodder.co.uk

For Norman Langer—Give my regards to Broadway.

CONTENTS

Author's Note

This book could be read as anti–established medicine. It is therefore important to state that if I personally were to experience extreme health symptoms, I would go to my doctor, but there is little else I would do that is traditional.

COUNTER CLOCKWISE

CHAPTER 1

Counterclockwise

What we need is not the will to believe, but the wish to find out.

—William Wordsworth

There's no way to turn back the clock or to fight the inevitable. We age and the vigor of youth becomes only a memory as we are ravaged by time. Chronic illnesses take their toll, our health and strength diminish accordingly, and the best we can do is graciously accept our fate. Once sickness is upon us, we give ourselves over to modern medicine and hope for the best. We can't intervene as time marches on. Or can we?

In the 1970s my colleague Judith Rodin and I conducted an experiment with nursing home residents.[1] We encouraged one group of participants to find ways to make more decisions for themselves. For example, they were allowed to choose where to receive visitors, and if and when to watch the movies that were shown at the home. Each also chose a houseplant to care for, and they were to decide where to place the plant in their room, as well as when and how much to water it. Our intent was to make the nursing home residents more mindful, to help them engage with the world and live their lives more fully.

A second, control group received no such instructions to make their own decisions; they were given houseplants but told that the nursing staff would care for them. A year and a half later, we found that members of the first group were more cheerful, active, and alert, based on a variety of tests we had administered both before and after the experiment. Allowing for the fact that they were all elderly and quite frail at the start, we were pleased that they were also much healthier: we were surprised, however, that less than half as many of the more engaged group had died than had those in the control group.

Over the next several years, I spent a lot of time thinking about what had happened. Our explanation was that the results were due to the power of making choices and the increased personal control it affords. Although we couldn't make an airtight case, subsequent research would bear out our original understanding. Our research had taken place at the beginning of what was later termed the "New Age" movement and well before mind/body studies were conducted in laboratories around the country. It raised a nagging question: "What is the nature of the link from the nonmaterial mind to the material body?" Examples of this connection are all around us. We see a rat and show signs of fear as our pulse races and sweat breaks out on our skin; we think about losing a significant other and our blood pressure increases; we watch someone vomit and we feel nauseous ourselves. While we easily see evidence of the connection, it's not well understood. Even we had been surprised: it seemed odd that simply asking people to make choices would result in the powerful consequences that our study showed. Subsequently, I realized that *making choices results in mindfulness, and perhaps our surprise was because of the mindlessness we shared with most of the culture.* I began to realize that ideas about mind/body dualism were just that, ideas, and a different, nondualist view of the mind and the body could be more useful. If we put the mind and the body back together so that we are just one person again, then wherever we put the mind, we would also put the body. If the mind is in a truly healthy place, the body would be as well—and so we could change our physical health by changing our minds.

The next question for me was one of limits. To what extent can the mind influence the body? If I smelled a fresh donut and imagined eating it, would my blood sugar rise? Would people fully convinced that their teeth are in excellent condition have healthier-looking X-rays at their annual checkups? Do men who become bald at a young age and thus see themselves as prematurely old test as older physiologically than men their age with a full head of hair? Do women who undergo cosmetic surgery and see a more youthful self in the mirror age more slowly? The questions may seem a bit "out there," but they were worth asking.

In 1979, several years after that initial investigation with plants and nursing home residents, it seemed natural to continue testing the question of limits with an elderly population. My students and I devised a study—which we would later come to call the "counterclockwise study"—to look at what effects turning back the clock psychologically would have on people's physiological state.[2] We would re-create the world of 1959 and ask subjects to live as though it were twenty years earlier. If we put the mind back twenty years, would the body reflect this change?

As with many ideas, at first it seemed extreme, but the more we thought about it, the more possible it became. We finally decided it was worth the effort. My students weren't quite as confident as I was because it wasn't your usual study, but they quickly got caught up in my excitement.

To start, we consulted leading geriatricians to find the definitive biological markers of age to measure our results. Astonishingly, we were told there were (and still are) none. Without knowing someone's chronological age, science cannot pinpoint how old someone is. To do our research, however, we needed ways to measure how old people were both before and after the retreat, so we determined which psychological and physical measures were the best bets to use. In addition to weight, dexterity, and flexibility, we planned to measure vision with and without eyeglasses, for each eye separately and together, as well as sensitivity to taste. We would give potential participants intelligence tests, to assess how quickly and accurately they could complete a series of paper-and-pencil mazes, and we would test their visual memory. We would also take photographs that we could later evaluate for the *appearance* of changes. Finally, they would each be asked to fill out a psychological self-evaluation test. All of these tests would help us select participants and give us a way to measure potential improvements at the end of the study.

We advertised the study in local newspapers and circulars, describing the research as a study on reminiscing, where people in their late seventies or early eighties would spend a week at a country retreat and talk about the past. To keep the study simple, we decided to use only one gender in order to make room assignments and other logistics easier. We chose to use men. We wanted men who were not ill and who would be reasonably able to participate in the activities and discussions we had planned for them. Word got out. Many younger people wanted to learn more about the study and how it might benefit their elderly parents. Those selected based on their telephone interviews came to the office to take the baseline physical and psychological tests.

The interviews were memorable. At our first meeting, I asked a man named Arnold to tell me about himself and especially how he felt about his health and physical condition. Unlike other adult children who brought their parents in, Arnold's daughter sat back and let him talk without interruption. He told me about his life and the wide range of activities he used to enjoy, both physical and intellectual. Now he never had enough oomph to do much of anything. He had given up reading because he could barely see the words on the page even with glasses. He no longer played golf because it was too disheartening to walk the course as slowly as he did. When he left the house, he invariably caught a cold no matter what the month or how much he bundled up. Food didn't taste good to him anymore, he said. This was as dismal a picture of his life as I could imagine.

Then, Arnold's daughter—whom I had been silently praising for her willingness to let her father speak for himself—spoke up and condescendingly said that Arnold was "prone to exaggeration."

Sadly, Arnold didn't object to his daughter's dismissal of his complaints.

I told him that I didn't know if anything would change as a result of the study, but he might have a good time for a week. He agreed to join us.

As we did more interviews and listened to the participants' complaints about their health and physical limitations, my doubts began to increase. Would we find positive results, and would they be worth the considerable effort of putting together and conducting the study? It was clear to me and my four graduate students that this was indeed a major undertaking, but given the work we had already done, we decided to go forward. We selected participants, divided them into two groups of eight—an experimental group and a control group—and set about putting in place our plans for the experiment.

My students and I traveled to several towns to find an appropriate site for our weeklong retreat. The right spot needed to seem timeless, with few modern conveniences. We eventually found an old monastery in Peterborough, New Hampshire, that was perfect. Our plan was to retrofit it so that it would "replicate" the world of 1959. The "experimental" group of participants would live there for a week going about their lives as though that year were the present. Every conversation and discussion was to be held in the present tense. We sent everyone an information packet in the mail with general instructions, an outline of the week's schedule (including meals, discussion groups about movies and politics of the time, and each evening's activities), and a floor plan of the retreat, marking the location of their room. We told research subjects not to bring any magazines, newspapers, books, or family pictures that were more recent than 1959. They were asked to write a brief autobiography as though it were 1959 and send photos of their younger selves, which we sent to all of the other participants.

The second group—the control group—went on a separate retreat held a week later. They were treated just like the first: they would be living in the same surroundings and enjoying activities and discussions about things that took place in 1959. But their bios were to be written in the past tense, their photos were of their current selves, and once at the retreat they would *reminisce* about the past and thus largely keep their minds focused on the fact that it was not 1959.

For both groups, we knew that if we were going to turn back the clock, we would have to do so convincingly. We carefully studied what daily life in 1959 was like. We learned the particulars of current political and social issues, the television and radio programs people watched and listened to, and the physical objects they would have encountered. It was difficult, but we were able to create a program for a week's worth of events in an environment that would indeed persuasively mimic the past for our participants.

When the experimental group participants were brought together for their trip orientation, we introduced the present-tense nature of their experience; we stressed that the best way to approach the study might not be through simple reminiscence. Rather, they should return as completely as possible in their minds to that earlier time. I remember the excitement of saying, "Therefore, we're going to a very beautiful retreat where we will live *as if* it were 1959. Obviously, that means no one can discuss anything that happened after September 1959. It is your job to help each other do this. It is a difficult task, since we are not asking you to 'act as if it is 1959' but to let yourself be just who you were in 1959. We have good reason to believe that if you are successful at this, you also will feel as well as you did in 1959." We told them that all of their interactions and conversations should reflect the "fact" that it was 1959. "It may be difficult at first, but the sooner you let yourselves go, the more fun you'll have," I said enthusiastically. A few men laughed nervously, one giggled in excitement, and a couple just shrugged cynically.

And so off we went to spend a week in the "nifty fifties," a time when an IBM computer filled a whole room and panty hose had just been introduced to U.S. women.

Once at the retreat, we met daily to discuss current events such as the 1958 ("last year" in the case of the experimental group) launch of the first U.S. satellite, Explorer 1; the need for bomb shelters; and Castro's advance into Havana. A talk on communism became very heated, as did a recap of the Baltimore Colts': 31–16 defeat of the New York Giants in the NFL championship game. We listened as Royal Orbit won the Preakness, watched Sgt. Bilko and Ed Sullivan on a black-and-white television, and shared our thoughts about "recent" books such as Ian Fleming's *Goldfinger*, Leon Uris's *Exodus*, and Philip Roth's

Goodbye Columbus. Jack Benny and Jackie Gleason made us laugh; Perry Como, Rosemary Clooney, and Nat "King" Cole sang on the radio, and we watched movies like *The Diary of Anne Frank, Ben Hur, North by Northwest*, and *Some Like It Hot*.

What happened? We noticed a change in behavior and attitude in both groups before the respective weeks were up. Indeed, by the second day everyone was actively involved in serving meals and cleaning up afterward. Despite their obvious and extreme dependence on relatives who initially drove them to Harvard's psychology department for interviews, they were all functioning independently almost immediately upon arrival at the retreat. After each weeklong retreat was over, we retested all participants and found that indeed, the mind has enormous control over the body. Both groups had been treated with respect, engaged in lively discussions, and experienced a week unlike anything in their recent past. Both groups also came out of the experience with their hearing and their memory improved. For better or worse—in most cases for better—they gained an average of three pounds each and the strength of their grip increased significantly. On many of the measures, the participants got "younger." The experimental group showed greater improvement on joint flexibility, finger length (their arthritis diminished and they were able to straighten their fingers more), and manual dexterity. On intelligence tests, 63 percent of the experimental group improved their scores, compared to only 44 percent of the control group. There were also improvements in height, weight, gait, and posture. Finally, we asked people unaware of the study's purpose to compare photos taken of the participants at the end of the week to those submitted at the beginning of the study. These objective observers judged that all of the experimental participants looked noticeably younger at the end of the study.

This study shaped not only my view of aging but also my view of limits in a more general way for the next few decades. Over time I have come to believe less and less that biology is destiny. It is not primarily our physical selves that limit us but rather our mindset about our physical limits. Now I accept none of the medical wisdom regarding the courses our diseases must take as necessarily true.

If a group of elderly adults could produce such dramatic changes in their lives, so too can the rest of us. To begin, we must ask if any of the limits we perceive as real do exist. For example, we largely presume that as we age our vision gets worse, that chronic diseases can't be reversed, and that there is something wrong with us when the external world no longer "fits" as it did when we were young.

Why is it that, as a society, we pay so much attention to our health and yet we know so little about achieving a healthy life? We read article after article in magazines. There are mountains of books and television shows devoted to improving our health; we are obsessed with health and fitness. Yet if we look carefully, psychology tells us that we are not attuned to our health at all. On the contrary, motivation and behavior often stand directly in the way of achieving the good health we seek. We need to try a more mindful approach, one that doesn't accept the limits we place on our health.

Mindful health is not about how we should eat right, exercise, or follow medical recommendations, nor is it about abandoning these things. It is not about New Age medicine nor traditional understandings of illness. It is about the need to free ourselves from constricting mindsets and the limits they place on our health and well-being, and to appreciate the importance of becoming the guardians of our own health. Learning how to change requires understanding how we go astray. The goal of this book is to convince you to open your mind and take back what is rightfully, sensibly, and importantly yours.

If One Dog Could Yodel

Most people believe that "always" and "never" are rarely appropriate ways of understanding human events. This belief is akin to the more scientific observation that what is true for the general case may not be true in any particular instance; with few if any exceptions, we cannot predict any particular outcome at any particular time. What may be true for most people most of the time matters less to us than what is true for any one of us at any particular time. If my leg needs to be amputated, the fact that most people survive the surgery is of little comfort.

Science has come a long way in providing answers to serious and important questions. Nevertheless, scientific data only speak to the general case, to what is generally true. Whether any particular medication or medical procedure is deemed effective is determined by a study of what works in a population that had the presenting problems under investigation. For practical reasons alone, all types of people—and their different body types, genetic makeup, lived experiences, and so on—are not equally likely to be among those studied. Every aspect of the investigation is a best guess at the time: which people to include as research subjects, which symptoms and in what combination to consider, which aspects of the procedure to focus on, and which measures to take are all based on choices made by the medical world. Because the task before medical science is enormous in its complexity and experiments cannot incorporate all the unknowns, it is with good reason that the findings of these studies are given in terms of probabilities—as general truths.

A perceptive reader might ask, "Why are your studies any different?" Much of my own research is designed to test possibilities, not to find what is descriptively true. If I can make one dog yodel, then we can say that yodeling is possible in dogs. The results of the counterclockwise study do not show us that everyone who talks about the past will show the same results. It does tell us, however, that it is *possible* to achieve these kinds of improvements, but only if we try.

Research in general tells us something about "most" people. Given that our concern is for what we, rather than what most people, should do, current medical practice alone cannot have a definitive answer. Medical science is not wrong or useless, but we as individuals are the keepers of some missing data. We need to learn how to integrate what the medical world knows to be generally true with what we know, or can find out, about ourselves.

If we spill a drop of red sauce on a white shirt, we easily will notice it. If the shirt were a busy plaid, we might not. Most of us are so disengaged from ourselves—stressed, depressed, overworked, and so on—that we look at ourselves and see plaid shirts. But that can change if we take note of what's new and different about the world and ourselves. When we notice new things, we become mindful, and mindfulness begets more mindfulness. The more mindful we become, the more we see ourselves as white shirts and the easier it is to find the red spot and remove it.

Attending to the world doesn't mean that we need to become hypervigilant. Our attention naturally goes to what is different and out of balance. If we allow it, we will begin to notice small signals without consciously searching or paying any particular attention to them. But first we need to open our minds to possibility. We all pay lip service to the idea that anything is possible. Yet whenever specific instances of "never-before" happenings present themselves, most of us reject the possibility out of hand. Can limbs regenerate? Can paralysis be reversed? Many of us who otherwise agree that anything is possible will respond no almost without thinking. Why don't we allow in practice what we profess to believe? One answer is that the mindsets we form from everyday experience close us off to possibility. It doesn't occur to

ethink much of what we learn about the world because we
d to learn mindlessly; it's not that we aren't paying attention
to whatever it is we are learning, it's that we aren't paying attention to the context in which we learn it. We don't consider that
what's true here need not be true over there. If we don't think to
think about our ideas, we can't update or improve them. It won't
occur to us to question how we know what we know, what facts
we base it on, and whether the science that produced those facts
is suspect. The hefty price for accepting information uncritically
is that we go through life unaware that what we've accepted as
impossible may in fact be quite possible.

Most people, including scientists, engage in hypothesis-
confirming behavior. Once we think we know something, we
search for information consistent with that belief. Seek and ye
shall find. If we searched for the opposite of what we believe to
be true, we would likely also find confirmation and in many
cases we could be better served. Social psychologists typically
do this by looking for interactions among variables, expecting
the effect in question to be true in some situations and not in
others. If we all did this more generally, we might discover something we didn't know or we might develop more nuanced beliefs.
When we simply search for confirmation of our beliefs, however,
we usually collect more evidence for the same hypothesis and potentially erroneous beliefs become harder to dispel. (It's even true
that experimenters investigating the phenomenon of hypothesis
confirmation have the same problem of seeking hypothesis confirmation.) We often find the source of our beliefs in conventional
wisdom and their proof in expert opinion. For example, we believe generally that alcohol is basically bad for us, and science—
expert opinion—believes that this is often the case. Doctors who
treat alcoholics confirm it. In many cases, it simply doesn't occur
to us to question either of these "truths." If we did, our trust in the

impossible might yield to a belief in possibility. Now we all know, for example, that red wine can actually be good for us.

The Psychology of Possibility

In most of psychology, researchers describe what is. Often they do this with great acumen and creativity. But *knowing what is and knowing what can be are not the same thing*. My interest, for as long as I can remember, is in what can be, and in learning what subtle changes might make that happen. My research has shown how using a different word, offering a small choice, or making a subtle change in the physical environment can improve our health and well-being. Small changes can make large differences, so we should open ourselves to the impossible and embrace a psychology of possibility.

The psychology of possibility first requires that we begin with the assumption that we do not know what we can do or become. Rather than starting from the status quo, it argues for a starting point of what we would like to be. From that beginning, we can ask how we might reach that goal or make progress toward it. It's a subtle change in thinking, although not difficult to make once we realize how stuck we are in culture, language, and modes of thought that limit our potential. For instance, we all use pithy expressions such as "We won't know unless we try," but we don't realize how misleading they can be. I maintain that we may not know even if we try, because when we try and fail, all we know is that the way we tried was not successful. We still do not know that it *can't* be.

When faced with disease or infirmity, we may find a way to adjust to what is. In the psychology of possibility, we search for the answer to how to improve, not merely to adjust.

For example, most of us believe that between the ages of forty and fifty, our eyesight will start to decline. Indeed, research has shown that while it may not happen to everybody, a loss of vision happens much of the time. But we too often mindlessly turn this probability into absolute fact. When we begin to have trouble reading we accept that our eyes have worsened and we adjust to the loss by getting glasses. I'm not suggesting that optometrists give us glasses when we physiologically don't need them. I'm not arguing that we don't need the glasses at this point. But if we didn't accept that our eyes were going to chronically get worse, they might not. If instead we thought that perhaps our eyesight could improve over time—be better than when it was at its best—we might develop ways to make that happen. Consider how the deaf come to see better just as the blind develop more acute hearing. Surely we can find that we see some things better than others. So it would make sense to ask why not try to see the less clear more clearly. We probably wouldn't even ask ourselves; we would just do it.

The second step toward embracing a psychology of possibility—using our eyesight as a continued example—is to try out different things without evaluating ourselves as we go along. If we squint when trying to read small print and we still have trouble, our self-esteem would not be particularly on the line. We would simply note whether or not the attempt was successful. With the same attitude, we would be more likely to notice other anomalies regarding our vision: perhaps that sometimes we can see the previously unseen and sometimes not, which could give us clues as to what was happening to our vision. In this way, the psychology of possibility is more positive, less evaluative, and more process-oriented than most personal and scientific research.

Pursuing possibility regarding our health may result in the desired end, but in addition, pursuing the psychology of possibility is itself empowering. It feels good to have a personal mission, it contributes to a more positive outlook in general, and it works against the idea that the rest of us are soon to follow suit and fall apart. As we actualize the possible, we may find out other interesting things about ourselves and the world. In exploring the "limits" of my vision, for example, I may see things around the house that I have too long ignored ("seeing them" through a fresh attempt to see them); I may notice that I need a new sofa (I notice frayed edges where I'd never bothered to look before) or that I am particularly fond of a painting on the wall that I ceased to appreciate years ago.

In the psychology of possibility, interpreting findings is also a different process. In descriptive or traditional psychology, the majority of subjects tested have to show an effect for us to conclude that the effect is real: a large number of monkeys would need to be able to speak clearly for us to conclude that monkeys can talk. In this new psychology, once we've ruled out experimenter error, only one participant is needed to prove that something is possible. If just one monkey spoke one real word, we'd have enough evidence to draw conclusions about primate communication abilities. Typically, participants who do not conform to the experimenter's hypothesis are seen as unwanted noise in the data. In my research, these exceptional cases become the focal point of the investigation.

In physics, concepts such as "dark energy" function as placeholders. It is acknowledged that we do not understand much about it, but science is well served to presume it exists. In psychology we do not have placeholders. The question is more often about why phenomena exist rather than if they can exist. Accordingly, psychology researchers look for mediating mechanisms to explain how they could be. If they can't be explained, the findings may be dismissed out of hand. For instance, many psychologists presume memory loss is a natural part of aging. An older person who doesn't have memory loss is seen as an anomaly instead of becoming a model for how we all might be. In the psychology of possibility, mediating mechanisms (or their absence) do not blindside us. The mission is to see if an outcome is possible first. After that, explanations for why and how can be pursued.

Too many of us believe the world is to be discovered, rather than a product of our own construction and thus to be invented. We often respond as if we and/or the world around us are fixed, even when we agree in theory that we are not. We might sit uncomfortably in the bathroom each day without realizing that we would feel better if we changed the height of the toilet. We lament that we can't paint until our broken wrist heals and never seriously consider painting with our nondominant hand. We don't go to the opera because of our glaucoma, when the experience of merely listening to the music could be extremely rich. There are many changes we would know how to make to feel better if it only occurred to us to ask. That's how strong the illusion of stability—mindlessness—is. We imagine the stability of our mindsets to be the stability of the underlying phenomena, and so we don't think to consider the alternatives. We hold things still in our minds, despite the fact that all the while they are changing. If we open up our minds, a world of possibility presents itself.

There are many cynics out there who are entrenched in their beliefs and hold dear their view of the world as fixed and predictable. There are also people who, while not cynical, are still mindlessly accepting of these views. A new approach to psychology and to our lives is needed because the naysayers—those who demand empirical evidence—are winning. It is they who have determined what's possible and what's achievable, to our collective detriment. If we suggest a possibility that seems far afield from what is currently known, the burden of proof is on us. Yet rather than ask "How could that be?" it makes just as much sense to ask "Why couldn't it be so?" What the naysayers know is only based on probabilities, which were deduced from a fixed view of what was studied. Just as we can't prove that something is so in advance of finding out, the naysayers can't prove that it is not possible. If I had never wondered about what is possible, I never would have conducted the counterclockwise study and never have witnessed the transformative power of our minds.

CHAPTER 2

Health, Unlimited

His situation was exacerbated by reading medical textbooks and seeking advice from doctors. The deterioration continued so smoothly he was able to deceive himself when he compared one day to the next—there was little difference. But when he asked for medical advice it seemed to him that everything was getting worse, and very quickly too. And yet he continued to consult the doctors, regardless. That month he went to another eminent specialist, and that eminence said almost the same as the first one but posed the questions slightly differently. The advice of this eminence only intensified Ivan Ilyich's doubts and fears. . . . The pain in his side kept wearing him down and seemed to be getting steadily more sustained and severe. The taste in his mouth grew more and more peculiar; it felt to him as though some revolting smell was coming out of his mouth, and his strength and appetite were both diminishing.

—Leo Tolstoy, *The Death of Ivan Ilyich*[1]

The world of medicine didn't have much to offer Ivan Ilyich. Not one of the celebrated doctors he consulted knew how to cure him, nor did they offer him much understanding or emotional support. They kept him busy with any number of regimens and medicines, but none of these proved to be effective. Tolstoy's story presents what many of us would imagine to be the worst possible picture of an illness: a patient helplessly caught in a downward spiral from an unknown and untreatable condition.

While there are many interpretations of the meaning of Ivan's struggle, one observation stands out to me: Ivan Ilyich wasn't a very good patient, however much the medical system failed him. He mindlessly gave himself over to the medical world, much the way Tolstoy described he had given himself over to the social and material world earlier in the story. Most of us do this, of course, but it's not a good approach to our well-being. As the physician and writer Jerome Groopman once remarked, "We doctors need you to help us to think better. We need you to question us and engage us from a position of knowledge about how and when we think well and how and when we go astray. . . . It's really hard to be a doctor. But it's much harder to be a patient."[2] Ivan Ilyich never took up that challenge.

If it's hard to be a patient, it's harder still because of the mindsets that we bring to health and disease. "The baby, assailed by eyes, ears, nose, skin, and entrails at once, feels it all as one great blooming, buzzing confusion," wrote William James in 1891, a line often quoted to endorse making life simple by reducing uncertainty.[3] Most of us embrace simplicity without hesitation, even as we moan that our lives could well be simpler still. We don't pay close attention to things we deem to be irrelevant, although we all have had the experience of finding out that the irrelevant can become critical down the road. We apply convenient labels to most everything we encounter, blinding ourselves to alternative ways of understanding that would have made just as much sense and could turn out be far more useful. We seek out certainty over a more nuanced understanding, only to feel frustration when even experts aren't able to be certain.

Ever since the counterclockwise study, my students and I have continued to research how our well-being is linked to our mindset. We recently conducted a study that looked into the question "If the life we live resembles that of a different age group, will we age like that group or be more similar to our own age cohorts?" We found that women who marry men much younger than they are live longer than average and those married to much older men die younger. The same is true for men, even as the average life expectancies are different. The psychologist Bernice Neugarten suggested we are deeply influenced by "social clocks"—that we gauge our lives by the implicit belief that there is a "right age" for certain behaviors or attitudes.[4] We reasoned that if we set our own social or biological clocks in accordance with our spouse's age, we change the game. In this way, the older spouse becomes "younger" and lives longer than expected, while the younger one becomes "older" and dies sooner than expected.

Other research has shown that women are less likely to die in the week before their birthday but more likely to die in the week after.[5] Men, on the other hand, are more likely to die in the week before and show no rise above normal the week after. The results suggest that women and men "package reality differently," in the words of David Jenkins, commenting on the research.[6] The packaging we create or the way we frame information for ourselves has real effects. For example, women tend to be hopeful in the lead-up to their birthdays and look forward to the celebration. It would appear that men do not care as much.

In a recent study of personality, aging, and longevity, my former student, psychologist Becca Levy, and her colleagues found that people's mindsets may contribute more to their health than the physiological factors we and our doctors typically focus on.[7] They looked at the life spans of a group of more than 650 people in Oxford, Ohio, who in 1975 had been asked to respond to positive and negative statements about aging. They could agree or disagree with thoughts such as "Things keep getting worse as I get older," "As you get older, you are less useful," and "I am as happy now as I was when I was younger." Scoring their responses allowed the participants to be categorized as holding either a positive or negative view of their health and aging.

In checking the records of the participants more than twenty years after the survey, Levy and her colleagues found that those who viewed aging more positively lived, on average, seven and a half years longer than those who were negative about it. Simply having a positive attitude made far more difference than any to be gained from lowering blood pressure or reducing cholesterol, which typically improve life span by about four years. It also beats the benefits of exercise, maintaining proper weight, and not smoking, which are found to add one to three years. In 1999, psychologists Heiner Maier and Jacqui Smith published a study of the relationship between mortality and seventeen indicators of psychological well-being, including intellectual ability, personality, subjective well-being, and social ability.[8] Using data from the Berlin Aging Study, which had collected information on the physical and psychological health of more than five hundred people in the early 1990s, they also found that dissatisfaction with aging was one of the principle factors in how long people live.

People read the results of studies such as this and think, "That's interesting, but that can't have much to do with me." The idea that our beliefs might be one of the most important determinants of our life span goes too much against the grain of what we "know" to be true. We have to put aside our mindless belief in what we "know" in order to understand that while we can know that something is, we cannot know that something cannot be. No science, no matter how sophisticated, can reveal that something is uncontrollable. At best, all that it can tell us is that something is indeterminate.

There is an important benefit in understanding the difference between an uncontrollable world and an indeterminate one. The fact that something has not happened doesn't mean it cannot happen; it only means that the way to make it happen is as yet unknown. We might never try to cure a disease if we believed that it was incurable or uncontrollable. The effort would be pointless. Most diseases medical science has conquered were at one time thought to be uncontrollable when they were really just indeterminate, and that change in attitude has made all the difference.

If our beliefs have influence on our well-being, surely we can learn to influence our beliefs. To begin to do so, we must make a critical choice. We must choose to believe that we have control over our health. There isn't a guarantee that we will always succeed, but if we are correct, we will have conquered the "uncontrollable." If not, we will find other rewards from the search itself. The greater loss, however, is if we choose not to believe. In that case, we have lost at least the rewards of having tried and more likely the opportunity to exercise meaningful control over our health.

Taking Control of Health

In more than thirty years of research, I've discovered a very important truth about human psychology: *certainty is a cruel mindset*. It hardens our minds against possibility and closes them to the world we actually live in. When all is certain, there are no choices for us. If there is no doubt, there is no choice. When we are certain, we are blind to the uncertainties of the world whether we recognize it or not. It is uncertainty that we need to embrace, particularly about our health. If we do so, the payoff is that we create choices and the opportunity to exercise control over our lives.

We don't often recognize how our mindsets limit us. Consider just a few of the common beliefs about health that many of us hold.

We are either ill or healthy. Just as we like to imagine that the mind and the body are separate, so we imagine that at any one point in time we are healthy or we are not, an attitude that brings unexpected consequences. When we are healthy, we imagine that we don't need to pay much attention to our health. When we are sick, we imagine that we should be able to find expert information that cures us. Whether that information comes from an expert or conventional wisdom, we expect that it will be a prescription for health. In both cases, we are favoring certainty over a more complex understanding of what health is.

The medical world knows best. Doctors surely know more about health in general than we do. But consider that just as surely, we ought to know more about ourselves than anyone else. Given the fact that no one can know us better than we can know ourselves, we need to take advantage of the medical world in association with the perspective we uniquely can offer.

Health is a medical phenomenon. It is not an exaggeration to say that we overmedicalize the world. It is rare that we experience sadness; instead we are depressed. If we problem-solve at night and our sleep is less than the "required" eight hours, we call ourselves obsessive or insomniac. Instead of taking responsibility for our choices, we call ourselves procrastinators, although every time we do something, there are other things that by necessity and definition we are not doing. Why do we see it as appropriate to label ourselves and what is the cost of doing so? We have mindlessly exchanged healthy experience for medicalizing our behavior, where almost everything becomes a medical condition or syndrome.

Challenge or difficulty becomes disability, and sensations become symptoms. In attributing so much of our experience to a medical condition, we limit our understanding of it (indeed, we abdicate the need to understand it in the first place since we believe that doctors understand these things better) and come to see that medical condition as affecting more of our lives than is warranted.

The way to regaining control of our health is through understanding the reasons we unknowingly give it up. Often when I lecture on mindfulness, I ask if anyone knows their cholesterol level. Someone with a fine bill of health usually waves an attention-getting hand. After he tells us his cholesterol level, I ask when it was last checked. The answer always varies, but it's typically at least a month old. "So," I respond, "you haven't eaten or exercised since? If you never get it checked again, you'll die a healthy person." My response always gets a laugh, but it's a serious observation. The medical world gives us numbers like cholesterol level, and we act as if they are unchanging—at least until our next visit to the doctor. Our health right now is not fixed by our past or defined by past experience.

The mindlessness of our approach to our health is remarkable in its backwardness. We ignore our health until we think we need to become health experts. Instead, we ought to attend to our bodies mindfully while being health learners.

Granting Permission—Mindlessly

We don't realize how mindless our interactions with the world and each other can become. It's common for us not to question even absurd information when it presents itself, because it fits some established belief or ingrained form of behavior.

In 1978, I conducted a study with my students Arthur Blank and Benzion Chanowitz in which we approached people in line to use a copy machine and asked if we could move ahead of them.[9] We sought permission through one of three requests: "May I use the Xerox machine?" "May I use the Xerox machine because I want to make copies?" or "May I use the Xerox machine because I'm in a rush?" As one might expect, permission was granted more when we used the second and third forms of request, since unlike the first, they gave the person ahead of us a reason for the request. What was interesting was that permission was granted equally to those two requests, even though asking to use the Xerox machine because I want to make copies is not much of a reason to allow me to move ahead in line. What else would I use it for? The "because I am in a rush" request had a better rationale for needing to move ahead, but it didn't result in convincing more people to agree to let us do so.

We concluded that people mindlessly agreed to the "because I want to make copies" request because it had the structure of a request containing a valid reason for moving ahead in line, if not the content. In other words, people were willing to grant permission so long as a reason was offered, no matter how inane the reason was. It seems silly, but we do much the same thing when we mindlessly accept a piece of information as fact, assume advice to be prescription, or grant that doctors know more about our health than we can. We aren't paying attention to content because we are mindlessly focused on form. While it doesn't matter all that much in minor social situations, it matters a great deal if our health is at stake.

The triumph of form over content is so ingrained in us that we rarely think to question a doctor's orders. Just as rarely does the medical world bother to request that we follow their "orders"; they just give them. It may be called advice rather than an order, but we are expected to go along with it without much questioning. And we do. While in the copying study an empty reason increased compliance, in the case of the doctor the implicit reason is "Because I am the doctor," or the explicit reason given is "This medication will reduce or eliminate the problem."

This is not to say that the medical world is not trustworthy. It is simply, but importantly, to say that the medical world is itself operating in uncertainty, no matter how cut-and-dried some physicians may make it seem. And it's important to note that the medical world is operating in enough uncertainty that it makes no sense to absent ourselves from the decision-making process regarding our health because of our own uncertainty.

Diagnosis: A Starting Point

Years ago a student of mine, Anne Benevento, and I did research on the effect of labels on our sense of competence, a phenomenon we called self-induced dependence.[10] In a series of experiments, we showed that titles such as "assistant" demonstrably undermine our abilities. To extrapolate, the same effect can take hold when we think of ourselves as patients who are less knowledgeable than doctors. We become, in fact, less able. Furthermore, when we relinquish control to others, we often have a hard time taking it back. We come to see ourselves as incompetent, even if we are not.

Diagnoses, for example, are labels. They tell us what certain sensations signify and how they ought to be interpreted. They tell us whether a series of experiences is chronic or congenital, whether a decline suggests a relapse or deterioration. They tell us what to expect and what to look out for, whether something is curable or incurable. They tell us if an ache is a symptom or a side effect or merely a sensation. They tell us what to fear and what we should learn to ignore or tolerate. Diagnoses are an essential component of medical decision making, but like any other label, they hold variable phenomena still and provide a single lens for

understanding multiple phenomena, not all of which may be reasonably attributed to the diagnosis. A diagnosis describes the av-
eraged experiences of many individuals, but it may not speak to a
single individual's experience at any one moment. In light of the
inherent variability in our bodies, sensations, and experiences, it
is misleading to put one label on the myriad manifestations of any
one diagnosis or to suggest that one label can sum up a person's
identity, condition, experiences, or potential. As with other labels,
diagnoses are best seen not as answers or explanations but as
starting points to guide the asking of additional questions. Too
often, though, diagnoses are taken at face value and hopes dashed
as a direct result.

We can become effective health learners only by questioning
the traditional ways we respond to medical information. We will
be ready to seek a new way if we recognize that doctors can only
know so much, that medicine is not an accumulation of absolute
truths, that incurable really means indeterminate, and that our
beliefs and most of the relevant external world are social constructions.

Diagnoses aren't unhelpful, and I am by no means suggesting
a hypervigilance that leads us to act like hypochondriacs. I am
suggesting paying mindful attention to our bodies so that we notice small changes that can be dealt with before larger problems
arise. Mindfulness is very different from vigilance. It is a soft
awareness marked by an absence of mindless attention to any
specific part of the body (or anything else, for that matter) that
prevents us from experiencing our fuller selves.

When we learn mindlessly, we look at experience and impose
a contingent relationship between two things—what we or someone else did and what we think happened as a result. We interpret that experience from a single perspective, oblivious to the
other ways it can be seen. Mindful learning looks at experience
and understands that it can be seen in countless ways, that new

information is always available, and that more than one perspective is both possible and extremely valuable. It's an approach that leads us to be careful about what we "know" to be true and how we learn it. At the level of the particular experience, each event is unique. Why then do we think we can learn from experience? That is, if events don't necessarily repeat themselves, what can one event teach us about a future event? What can one pain on one occasion teach us?

I was on a walk with two friends and one recounted a horrible experience she had had several years earlier. I missed the reason for her mishap but tuned in when she said she had been standing on top of a porcelain toilet. It cracked, she slipped, and the porcelain nearly severed her leg, resulting in 106 stitches. She said she'd learned her lesson. I asked her what the lesson was, and she replied, "Don't stand on porcelain toilets." Perhaps, but I suggested that the lesson could be any of the following: "Be more cautious," "Don't try to fix things yourself," "Make sure you're not alone when attempting something new," "Don't attempt anything new," "Wear heavy clothes when fixing things," "Don't be afraid to try new things because the body is amazing the way it heals itself," "I can take a hit and not be defeated," or "Lose weight so toilets can hold me." I could have gone on indefinitely, but I valued our friendship, so I stopped there. It's not that her response was wrong, but that it was only one way to view the experience. Rather than try to learn from experience, we might be better off to experience learning.

Experience can be a feeble teacher. How do we learn when we think we are learning from experience? We look back at the experience—an experience that could be understood in countless ways—and impose a relationship between two things even though many other relationships could have been constructed. Once we have the relationship in mind we look for confirmations and eliminate alternative understandings. So experience too often "teaches" us what we already know. Sometimes yesterday's progress is today's failure. We try walking on a broken leg that is healing and we're doing fine, and then we see we've pushed ourselves too far and the next day we have to take it easier. We could have understood our past experience to lead us to give up, take it easy, or try harder. Becoming a health learner requires us to be open to all the lessons we can take from the world. It also demands that we attend to small things as well as big ones and to appreciate that small changes can, over time, prove significant. Often something feels impossible even though we recognize that it is not. It may be overwhelming to think about losing fifty pounds. It is the rare person, I think, who would be overwhelmed with the thought of losing an ounce. We need to find the ounce of cure.

CHAPTER 3

Variability

One morning, as Gregor Samsa was waking up from anxious dreams, he discovered that in bed he had been changed into a monstrous verminous bug. He lay on his armour-hard back and saw, as he lifted his head up a little, his brown, arched abdomen divided up into rigid bow-like sections. From this height the blanket, just about ready to slide off completely, could hardly stay in place. His numerous legs, pitifully thin in comparison to the rest of his circumference, flickered helplessly before his eyes.

"What's happened to me," he thought. It was no dream.

—Franz Kafka, "The Metamorphosis"

People aren't all that observant, although we think we are. We see what we expect to see, even to the point that we don't notice things that others clearly do. Sometimes it's because our expectations blind us to the world; other times it may be that we're afraid to notice change, even if the change isn't nearly as dramatic as being turned into a giant insect.

What we have learned to look for in a situation determines mostly what we see. At some point every semester I ask students in my seminar if I have time to tell them a story before going on to the day's discussion.

They look at their watches and say, "Sure, we have time."

I then ask them what time it is and most look again. Shouldn't they know what time it is, given that they just looked at their watches? The surprising answer is no, they shouldn't. The first time they looked they weren't really looking at what time it was; they were looking to see if there was enough time left before the class ended. It is not surprising that they didn't know the time. If we look for one thing, we may well miss another. While our expectations help us see, they also blind us to what we don't expect.

Consider the difference between a traditional analog watch and a digital one. A digital watch shows us the time most clearly, but all it displays is the time. An analog watch tells us "almost," "just past," "soon it will be," et cetera. In some ways it gives us more conditional information. Conditional information brings advantages, especially in that it leads us to notice variability. Noticing variability is the key to mindfulness. If I see that information changes, I'm in a better position to ask important questions about the changes, such as "When?" and "Why now and not then?"

For a researcher, variability is typically a curse. It can mean the difference between a publishable study and one that goes straight to the file cabinet. Essentially, researchers test their hypotheses, be it a drug treatment or assessing the effectiveness of ukulele instructions, by seeing whether it can improve conditions enough so that they can notice a difference beyond that which occurs by chance or "natural" variability. If I tested a drug to make people taller and everyone who got the drug got taller, and no one got taller who didn't get the drug, it would be easy to see the effectiveness of the treatment (though not the side effects). Rarely, however, are things so straightforward. The more variability there is in the conditions of the experiment, the harder it is to see if the drug is effective. If some people in both groups grew but the drug group got a little taller on average, the drug may or may not have resulted in a statistically significant difference. If not, the paper is not publishable and the drug—assuming there might have been a market for it—will not be easy to promote.

Recall the study with Judith Rodin that I described in Chapter 1, in which we wanted to see if nursing home patients could be made more engaged and improve their well-being if they were given the responsibility of taking care of a plant. One of our measures of the effectiveness of the experiment was a series of ratings of the participants' psychological well-being by the nurses who cared for them. Both day and evening nurses were asked to rate each nursing home resident. From a research perspective, it would have been perfect if they all reported the same thing. Glancing at the data, however, it appeared that some participants were seen as doing fine by one nurse and not very well by another. Some of them were reported as better in the morning and some were better at night. Was this variability significant enough to hide the effect of our treatment? The nurses' ratings of residents turned out to be close enough to each other to allow us to conclude that our hypothesis was correct and to publish the results, but a lingering question for me was whether the variability was actually among the nurses (that is, different nurses saw the same person differently) or whether the residents themselves changed from morning to night, so anyone would have noticed the change. As we will see, these alternatives—we are different from each other, and we are different from ourselves at different times and in front of different people—have important implications for our health.

Reversing Zeno's Paradox

At some point in school, many of us have had to confront Zeno's Paradox. I believe that Zeno must have been a pessimist. In one of the better-known examples of his paradoxes, we learn that if you always cover half the distance between where you are and where you want to be, you're never going to get there. In other words, if I'm two feet from a water fountain and always traverse half the distance to it, I'll never get a drink.

Ever the optimist in the eyes of others but the realist in my own, I've found a simple, positive use of this thinking that I call Reverse Zeno's Strategy. It states that there is always a step small enough from where we are to get us to where we want to be. If we take that small step, there's always another we can take, and eventually a goal thought to be too far to reach becomes achievable. One moment in the counterclockwise study provided me with a very clear example of this approach.

When all of the preparations for the retreat were in place, the participants met me and my graduate students in the parking lot of Harvard's William James Hall, where the psychology department is located. After they said their goodbyes to their families, we told them to get on the bus we had arranged to take them to the retreat. As I watched them hobbling—in some cases, almost being carried—to the bus I began to wonder again about what I had gotten into, but soon enough all were aboard and we were on our way.

As we traveled, we listened to music from the 1950s, including Nat "King" Cole singing "Mona Lisa," Johnny Ray's "Cry," and Hank Williams's "Your Cheating Heart." (To appreciate the effort it took to make the tape, go back in time to before the Internet existed. My students had scoured music stores in search of the appropriate music to record on the tape ourselves, a task they found more difficult since they knew little about 1950s music and didn't much like it.) As we rode, some of the men quietly watched the scenery out their windows while others chatted with the person sitting next to them.

The trip was uneventful, which led me to return to being excited about the week ahead. When we reached the retreat, my students made a quick exit to go pick up some equipment we would need for the week but hadn't yet set up. As soon as they were gone, I realized that I was alone with eight elderly men and just as many suitcases. The question of how the suitcases would get to their rooms hung in the air. My students weren't there to act as bellboys and the thought of being a "bell-professor" was totally unappealing, so I announced that each of them would be responsible for his own luggage. At first quietly surprised, they began to express their discomfort at the thought of carrying a heavy suitcase: "I haven't carried a bag for over a decade." "There must be a bellboy."

Not to worry, I told them. I suggested that if they couldn't take their suitcase to their room directly, they should do so slowly, moving it a few feet at a time toward their room. If that was too hard, then move it a few inches at a time. I also suggested that they could unpack their suitcase right there and bring each article one at a time to its final destination to lighten the load. A couple of them briefly winced but, to my relief, no one seemed to find any more reason to object. Although the incident was unplanned, right from the start they began to feel that this experience would be different from the overprotected way most of them were used to being treated.

Each of them took me up on the suggestions I had made that suited them best. A few managed to carry their suitcases directly into the building and to their rooms. Most carried them a short distance, stopped to rest, and then began again. I could see from their faces, however, that the task was actually empowering. Although they would not have thought themselves capable, and some literally carried their suitcase up one step at a time, they all managed to get their luggage to their rooms without help. As I watched, the ancient proverb came to mind: "A journey of a thousand miles begins with a single step." In Reverse Zeno's Strategy, the single step is defined differently—halfway between where we are and where we want to be.

People have a tendency to see what is and to assume that is what must be. If there is always a small enough step that we can take toward our goal, however, it suggests that the limits we often assume as necessary may be of our or our culture's making in even more dramatic cases. Years ago, while consulting to a nursing home, I worked with an elderly woman whose upper body was paralyzed. I asked her, "What can't you do that you wish you could?" She explained that she wished she could blow her own nose, as she found needing someone to do this for her humiliating.

I began to work with her, asking her to move her arm six inches from her side toward her nose. She couldn't do it, but we kept lowering the distance until there was slight movement. After much work and many steps, she was able to blow her own nose.

Skeptics will cry out, "Her paralysis was probably misdiagnosed, and so there isn't any proof that there's always a step one can take." To the first, my response is that yes, there may have been an error in her diagnosis, which meant that trying to get her to move her arm was exactly the right thing to do. Moreover, how many of us are similarly misdiagnosed? To the second I would reply that even if our efforts had not worked, it would not mean that for anyone else the attempt would not work. Negative results only mean we have no evidence for a hypothesis, which is a very different thing from saying we have evidence against it. By assuming misdiagnosis whenever the "impossible" happens, we rob ourselves of the chance to question the original presumption.

We can all say we believe in the possibility of improvement, but unless we really do, we won't find it. That is, we are more likely to find it if we look than if we presume it cannot be found. All told, we can accept the idea that we have no control and be correct or incorrect, although life is meaningless in the first case and wasted in the latter. But if we accept that we have control and are incorrect in any one instance, again, we can never be sure we won't find a way in the future and will reap the benefits of the search. And if we are correct, we have conquered the so-called uncontrollable.

Why try to help ourselves if we have a disease that's uncontrollable? There wouldn't be much point. Remember, virtually every disease medicine has conquered was at one time thought to be uncontrollable, and again, it took someone to think it indeterminate to find out how to conquer it.

Even scientists often make a mistake with this distinction. One notices a phenomenon and creates a theory to explain it. Then the theory is tested and voilà, the phenomenon occurs and the theory is taken to be true. One problem with working backward like this is that often these theories are like a house of cards: the theory is the first layer and subsequent layers are made up of facts that fit the theory but could have also been used to explain alternatives. Because the theory predicts the phenomenon, the phenomenon is then assumed to be more stable than it may be.

These confirmations do not mean that things could not be different. Years ago, there was a theory of disengagement to explain why elderly adults are typically less engaged in the world than younger people are. Research was undertaken and it was found that, yes indeed, elderly adults typically disengage—the observation that led to the theory in the first place. Because we had a theory leading us to expect elderly adult disengagement, it took some time for people to understand that disengagement needn't result from getting older. We have no shortage of such theories when it comes to our health. We believe there are known limits to how fast we can run, how much we should eat or not eat, how quickly our bones can heal, or how much sleep is necessary to perform effectively, to mention just a few.

The Googliasaurus

Everything is the same until it is not. Tightly woven ideas and theories may be fabrications that make it hard to see how things could be otherwise. Scientists elaborate on theory with a series of concatenated probabilities to the point that it becomes very difficult to take accepted truth apart in the face of so much "supporting" data. For example, while we all have a pretty good picture of what dinosaurs looked like, clearly no one has ever actually seen one. At first, a few bones were found and a picture of dinosaurs was constructed based on someone's view of how they fit together. Then more bones were found and it was easier to put together the picture of other dinosaurs once we had a starting point. Now imagine that a new and different set of bones were found and scientists began creating a picture of what would become googliasaurus, where the bones made a reasonably complete image. After it was finished, imagine that a new bone was found that didn't fit the prior conception of the googliasaurus. How many new, previously missing pieces that don't fit would have to be found before we remade entirely our conception of a googliasaurus?

We might "know," for instance, that certain brain injuries create "irreversible" brain damage, and accept that as fact. But if we asked how we could reverse "irreversible" brain damage, we would seek out information different from what we now examine when we take these labels as hard-and-fast truths and merely test existing theories. And so our medical conditions appear more and more as they have been defined by the research behind them.

Attending to Variability

In 1961, Yale psychologist Neal Miller suggested that the autonomous nervous system, which controls blood pressure and heart rate, could be trained just like the voluntary system, which allows us to raise or lower our arm and other deliberate acts.[1] His suggestion was met with a great deal of skepticism. Everyone knew that the autonomous system was just that, autonomous and beyond our control. Yet his subsequent work on biofeedback—which makes autonomic processes such as heart rate visible by hooking people up to monitors—found that people could be taught to control them. If we recognize that we can control the unseen, controlling the visible can seem a more doable task. Once we learn to pay attention to variability, that is, to notice change, we are in a better position to ask what the reason for the changes we observe might be and to ask what we can do to control the change.

My colleague Laura Delizonna, Ryan Williams, and I recently conducted research to see if people could be taught to regulate their heart rate after focusing their attention on how it varies.[2] We asked participants to record their heart rate by taking their pulse over the course of the day for a week, although we set different conditions for each of four groups. People in what we called the "stability group" measured their heart rate upon going to sleep and at first awakening every day for a week. We expected that this group would be likely to see their heart rate as reasonably stable, with little change from one measurement to the next. A "moderate attention to variability group" was asked to measure their heart rate twice a day, at different times each day that we predesignated for them. We expected that they would see a greater degree of variation in their rate.

The "high attention to variability group" was told to measure their heart rate every three hours, which would most likely ensure a great deal of variability in the recorded numbers. In addition, we instructed this group to record the activity they were engaged in at the time of the reading and to pay attention to the degree to which their heart rate differed from previous measurements as a way of getting them to be more mindful of the variability. Finally, a control group of participants did not monitor their heart rate; they were simply asked to monitor their activities for the week.

Beforehand, all the participants completed a brief questionnaire about one's ability to control their heart rate, completed a test of their mindfulness, and were sent home. They returned to the lab after a week of monitoring, and after gathering their data we gave them the surprise task of first raising and then lowering their heart rate. No one was instructed on how to control their heart rate; they were just asked to use their mind to change their heart rate without changing their muscle tension or breathing.

Both the "stability group" and the "moderate attention to variability group" weren't very good at increasing their heart rate, but the "high attention to variability group," the more mindful group, did significantly better. The difference was small but meaningful. The control group, interestingly, tended to decrease their heart rate even as they were attempting to increase it. Those who scored highest on the mindfulness scale, regardless of the group to which they were assigned, were more successful at raising their heart rate and exercised greater control over heart rate regulation. We don't know exactly how they did it, but our concern was with whether mindful awareness would enable them to find a way.

Instructing people to notice variability and biofeedback both provoke mindfulness. While they are similar, there are important ways attention to variability is different. Biofeedback assists a person to gain control over autonomous processes by employing an external device, such as a heart rate monitor, to make the process accessible. Biofeedback is a very important tool that deserves to be more fully explored, but attention to variability need not rely on external devices, nor need it be focused on solely biological phenomena. The effects of our attention to variability can be very general, bringing physiological responses, emotions, and behaviors within our control. Probably the most important difference between the two is that in biofeedback experiments, people are instructed how to change their bodily process. In our study, the "high attention to variability" group, told to notice change, was simply exposed to conditions that would foster such learning.

The Illusion of Stability

If attention to variability can be effective in such an "uncontrollable" process as heart rate, it may be effective in situations where our control is even more apparent—if we choose to notice, as in a disease such as asthma. Although we lead ourselves to believe that chronic conditions such as asthma become "manageable" as we learn to approach them in a consistent, predictable fashion, all diseases and the symptoms they present vary to some degree day by day if not minute by minute. An asthmatic's first task should be to recognize that the most stable thing about her disease is her mindset about it. The shortness of breath she experiences is never really the same as it was the last time or the time before that, although the differences too often go unnoticed.

Medical devices such as inhalers foster this illusion of stability. The inhaler doles out much the same amount of medication regardless of our need; it is not calibrated to lead us to consider how much we actually need at this particular moment. If an asthmatic noticed that his current episode is not as bad as—or is worse than—the last, it likely occurs to him to ask why that is so. It might be that when he has an episode while visiting Jane, he doesn't need the inhaler, but he needs an extra dose at Stephen's house.

With that information, he begins to figure out what tends to trigger his asthma and how to control these episodes better. Perhaps he shouldn't spend time at Stephen's anymore, or he might investigate what is different about each environment. Recognizing that there are distinct external circumstances that give rise to our symptoms is itself empowering, and using that information sends us on a self-rewarding, mindful journey in search of a solution.

All types of diseases and psychological processes are just as open to our attention. Consider depression. Typically, when we are depressed we have little or no desire for the company of others or interest in looking for activities that might break the spell of depression. We tend to feel that no person and no distraction can help and that engaging might even make us feel worse. Our answer is to retreat even further and avoid a change in circumstance, lest it prove to worsen our condition. Familiarity is comforting and we cling to the familiar to avoid the possibility of stress. When we're depressed, we take comfort in holding our routines still, even as they induce and reinforce our disengagement. The mindset of depression is such that people who are depressed often believe that they are always depressed, that their depression is a constant factor in their lives.

There is a different approach. When we grow depressed we tend to imagine that we are falling back into a familiar and even necessary condition, one no different from the other episodes of depression we've experienced. We don't consider that there are surely differences in our present circumstances or look to identify them. Our first experience of anything will be different from the tenth if we consider it clearly. One instance of depression may have needed a significant provocation; the next time perhaps all we needed was a subtle cue to bring it on. If we notice the differences between these bouts of depression, we have a chance to cope in a more successful way. One reason people come to see being depressed as a constant condition is that when we are content we don't check in with ourselves to see how we feel. We simply feel fine and go about living without gathering evidence about our feelings. When we grow depressed, we tend to ask why we are unhappy and gather evidence to support our depression. Thus, when we are depressed we ask why, and when we're happy we don't ask. As a result, when we become depressed we don't have complete information about our mental state and we have little evidence supporting our happiness, which allows us to imagine we're always depressed.

What would happen if we were encouraged to notice how our depression right now was different from the way it felt yesterday? We would become more mindful about our mental state. When we use a single attribution, "depressed," for our feelings, we are retreating into that term's familiar and mindless meaning. We feel less than alive, in part or whole, because we are not living. We're only existing. Now imagine if science led us to understand that there isn't a single kind of depression but rather five or more similar but distinct kinds of depression and that it was our job to figure out which kind we had. Let's say that we were told by doctors that we might experience more than one of them, and that we might have one kind of depression in the morning and another one in the evening, or even vacillate among a few of them throughout the day. Now, instead of a single-minded mindless focus on ourselves—the hallmark, I believe, of depression—we would be mindfully focused. The result of this search, ironically, might actually reduce our depression.

Confronting Stability

There are several reasons that we cling to the illusion of stability to the extent that we do. First, although we recognize on some level that the world around us is always changing, we are oblivious to the fact that we mindlessly hold it still. When we are mindful, we notice. When we are mindless we "are not there" to notice that we are not there.

Second, from the moment we are born we are presented with absolute facts rather than situated ones. We aren't taught that distinctions such as young and old or healthy and unhealthy are social constructions and that their meaning depends on context. We are conditioned to learn about and see the world as a set of facts, such as $1 + 1 = 2$. The world is far more subtle than such facts allow, and we should have learned that $1 + 1 = 2$ only if we are using the base 10 number system, but that it equals 10 if the number system is base 2, and that $1 + 1 = 1$ if we are adding one wad of chewing gum to one wad of chewing gum.

The educational system forgoes that more nuanced approach in favor of certainty. It simplifies and makes the world seem more predictable than it is. And so we educate ourselves into mindlessness. As psychologist Silvan Tomkins often noted, some of us believe the world is to be discovered, while others believe it is to be invented.[3] There are great rewards to be had by "discovering" the "truth" and knowing these "truths" that provide incentives for us to cling to the illusion of stability. The stable, consistent world we accept mindlessly isn't the one we live in. One person's depression is different from another's and different from itself on different occasions whether we choose to notice these differences or not. Searching out the nature of our depression would be engaging, and that engagement may be mutually exclusive with feeling depressed.

Consider how we might mindfully approach interacting with a spouse who has a diagnosis of dementia. As many will agree, few people, if any, will manifest symptoms every minute of every day, which could lead us to ask whether people are demented when they do not show any symptoms. Putting that important but sticky question aside, we can still take advantage of the moments of lucidity. The occasional lucid moment is one of the heartbreaking things about dementia—the person we know and love is still in there somewhere. Recognizing that the diagnosis is only a probability could lead us to look more closely at those times when our spouse is more connected. (For those convinced that there might not be any lucid moments, consider, perhaps, the period just before falling asleep or right after a meal.) With this approach, we win by being more mindful in our interaction with the person, and he wins by getting mindful attention. Shouldn't we have the chance to cherish "sane" moments? Consider if a nursing home adopted this strategy, for example. Staff could look for variability in residents, family could be instructed to do so also, and even the resident could be brought into the process. Not only could they attend to each other but each could be tuned in to variability in self, staff, and family. It offers us a much more positive approach.

Some family members already do this. They look for the smallest signs of difference day to day and realize that therein lies hope for connection and continued relationship. When I've observed this happening, I find it both interesting and sad if people make the smallest distinctions only at this point in their loved one's life instead of having attended to them throughout their relationship.

The result of this mindful attention should be an increase in satisfaction, both direct and indirect. It is direct in that mindful attention makes our spouse feel cared for and seen. People are loath to accept statements about themselves when such statements are prefaced with the implied or explicit assertion that they always or never do something. We don't like to be stereotyped. We feel cared for when we are seen for who we are right now. The only way that can happen is for people to notice the vicissitudes in our behavior. Satisfaction improves indirectly in that mindful relationships are more satisfying. In fact, in recent research my student Leslie Coates Burpee and I found that even intimate relationships are more rewarding when they are characterized by mindfulness.[4] In a relationship, when I am mindful I'm likely to notice the subtle differences in your behavior and feelings, and you notice the same for me. I'm likely to make sense of your behavior given the particular circumstances you are in instead of making global attributions for what you do. If we are each mindful in our relationship, we're more likely to see each other's behavior from the actor's perspective. So I may see you as spontaneous instead of impulsive, consistent and stable rather than rigid.

After my grandmother was diagnosed as senile many years ago, I was surprised that a person who appeared as normal as she did could receive such a diagnosis. She seemed fine to me whenever we were together, and so that was the way I treated her. I felt lucky that we had that much more meaningful time together. First I thought the diagnosis was wrong. Then years later I became aware that people who are diagnosed as having dementia have lucid moments. Then I understood that a meaningful relationship with someone who is so diagnosed is still possible. And finally I came to the question of what is behind the lucid moments. If we ask that question, might we find ways to increase the frequency of such moments?

There are unintended results of ignoring what is happening in the moments when symptoms of any disease disappear or lessen. If we mindlessly expect them to reappear undifferentiated, we are likely to group experiences as similar even though they may be better understood differently. For example, if I have arthritis and experience some back pain, I may overlook the fact that my mattress needs to be changed. Instead I presume all my pains are the result of the arthritis. If I can see some details close up without glasses, what does it mean to say I have poor vision? Am I dyslexic when I'm reading a short passage without problem? We are not our disorders, and we shouldn't be defined or constrained by them.

I was playing cards with my eighty-eight-year-old father last week. He remembered every card I picked up and skillfully used that information to win the game. We later went to a pool, where he did his exercises, remembering how many laps he had done and how many more he needed to do. Later that evening he told me that he was having memory problems. When I asked him what sorts of things he was forgetting, he wasn't specific. He knew he had forgotten a few things here and there, and he just accepted that memory problems must be memory problems. Why did he not differentiate between his problems? Why should I accept that I am nearsighted when I can occasionally see what I'm not supposed to be able to see (those times I bother to look)?

Solutions tend to come when we are specific about problems. I told my father to write down, if he could, the types of things he couldn't remember, to see if a pattern emerged. My guess was that, at least some of the time, he was "forgetting" things he didn't much care about and probably hadn't commited to memory in the first place—a necessary precondition to forgetting. If that was the case, he could be a lot easier on himself, or he could come to care about remembering them and thus be more likely to remember. He might even work at trying to improve his memory for such things, which is not as daunting a task as trying to improve memory more generally. Most of us forget specific information, but most aids to memory are general and thus limited in their usefulness. My father remembered a great number of things throughout the day, yet he focused on the fact that he forgot a few.

We are more likely to remember information that is meaningful to us than facts that are irrelevant to our daily lives. In one of our early studies, my colleagues and I provided incentives to nursing home residents to increase their mindfulness.[5] We gave the experimental group chips that could be exchanged for gifts every time they found out and remembered information we had requested, such as when certain activities would take place and nurses' names. Because they wanted the gifts, the information we asked them to track now mattered to them. We ran the experiment for three weeks before we took our measures to see if the intervention had been effective. We found improvements in memory and concluded that when remembering mattered, memory improved. On the last day, we administered several tests of cognitive ability, including one that asked them to describe their roommates and another that asked them to find novel uses for a familiar object. We found the group that was more mindful outperformed the other groups in the "new use" portion of the program, and when asked they were able to give more detailed descriptions of their roommates and their rooms although we didn't ask them to take note of either. Remarkably, this memory intervention also resulted in an increase in longevity. In our follow-up study, we found that only 7 percent of the mindful group had died compared to more than four times that in the comparison groups.

The common view is that long-term memory remains intact

at short-term memory diminishes: older adults often
ble remembering the name of someone they just met
no trouble telling detailed stories about their past. But
v that what is remembered is that which is meaningful
(regardless of age) is consistent with recent work in the field of
neuroscience. In studying memory, University of Michigan psychologists Derek Nee, Marc Berman, Katherine Sledge Moore,
and John Jonides found support for the view that memory is uni-
tary and little or no support for the long-held distinction between
long-term and short-term memory.[6] A new view of memory derived from such evidence may lead us to believe that memory
as we age may be less diminished than previously believed. If it's
the case that we are more likely to remember things that are
meaningful, it may well be that the old just happen to live in a
world created for younger adults and therefore one less personally relevant.

We have four possible ways of looking at the world. We could
always respond the same way to different things, we could
respond differently to things that are the same, we could respond the same way to the same things, and we could respond
differently to different things. What we don't keep in mind,
however, is that it is we who are creating the similarities and
differences. We tend to deal with the world around us at an
intermediate level of specificity. We observe a table. More generally, it is a piece of furniture. More specifically, it is a certain kind of table. Unless we are in the furniture business or
need to furnish a new home, for many of us a table remains a
table. But all tables are in some ways different. Change its
location—move a side table to function as a coffee table—and
the same table can become something very different. By expecting things to stay the same, we give up the chance to mindfully
notice or create subtle differences. We needn't. We could intentionally look for differences and choose whether to respond

differently or not. At the level of the specific, nothing is ever the same.

ADHD is taken as a generalized disability that impairs attention, along with learning, memory, and other high-level functioning. Yet virtually everything we do requires some degree of attention, and those diagnosed with ADHD are able to pay attention to many things. What would happen if instead of focusing on having the general problem, we paid attention to the specifics? Exactly when do I have trouble paying attention—mornings, evenings, weekdays, holidays? To exactly what do I have trouble paying attention—directions to doctors' offices or names of new acquaintances? Do I have trouble on these occasions and not on others because I don't really care about the information, I'm stressed, or I don't like being told what to do?

Attention to variability in our wants, needs, talents, and skills can result in the greater well-being we seek. Holding things still because we think we know leads us figuratively and literally to be blind to what needs improvement. A small growth, a change in breathing, a change in the color of our urine—these things too often go unnoticed unless the change is blatant. When we do notice the change, sometimes we don't want to confront it because we feel helpless. But these are signs that something needs attention. And these signs—the first change—appear much sooner than is now recognized. This blindness is not restricted to those of us who are not medical doctors. Physicians too miss minor deviations that could be meaningful.

We should take an interpersonal view of our health care whenever possible. You help me notice the external factors that seem to co-vary systematically with my symptoms and I notice them for you. Ultimately, the responsibility is still the individual's, but like therapists who point these things out to us, so too can our doctors, significant others, close friends, or relatives. Consider what would happen regarding an elderly parent in this regard. Adult children often feel helpless when trying to deal with their aging parents. Not infrequently they infantilize them and overprotect them. We often forget that whether or not a parent wants to wear a hearing aid, for example, is still her choice, not ours. Some older people may not want to hear what their children or nurses have to say. I have a friend whose liberal Democratic great-aunt would turn off her hearing aid when she and her arch-Republican husband set off from Boston to drive to the town where they voted. More important, hearing, like most everything else, is not likely to go away all at once, nor is our ability to hear the same for all types of sound and in all types of environment. A lack of interest may masquerade as a hearing loss. If we were to notice the distinctions in our parents' ability to hear—the times and conditions when their loss-is particularly great and when it is not—two things happen. First, we feel useful. Second, our parent may find the information useful. But most of us don't make these distinctions. Instead, we see them as experiencing a general loss, make unhelpful comments about their inability to hear, and shout when we may not have to.

Noticing differences is the essence of mindfulness. Don't imagine, however, that all this noticing need be exhausting and leave little time for anything else. Mindfulness is actually energizing, not enervating.

CHAPTER 4

The Social Construction of Health

We don't see things as they are, we see them as we are.

—Anaïs Nin

Suitcases in hand, all eight elderly men eventually made it to their respective rooms. While the rooms were not fancy, each man had his own room, and each room was decorated in a timeless fashion with an occasional object, like a piece of china or a vase, that was identifiable as from the 1950s. These details came as a surprise to our participants, as many thought they would basically be spending the week in a nursing home.

Until you spend time in a nursing home, it's hard to imagine what living in one is like. The doors to individual rooms remain open at all times, everything is done for you and on a schedule that you didn't choose—meals, when to shower, and where you can and cannot go are all out of your control.[1] When I first began working with elderly patients in nursing homes, I was saddened by what I saw: people sitting around with little to do and no choice regarding virtually any aspect of their lives. When I asked why the doors to their rooms were open, I was told that it was a fire hazard to close them. I asked when the last time was that they had a fire and was told, "Never."

The rooms at the retreat we chose afforded our participants all the privacy and personal responsibility they'd had twenty years earlier. They not only had choices at meals but were asked to participate in the preparation and clean-up. This week was going to be something different for them. Although we ensured their safety and watched carefully, they were essentially on their own.

Remember, when we designed the counterclockwise study, we tried to find the best measures to include to see if we could reverse or retard aging, but we came up short. We called several of the leading geriatricians around the country and asked, "If we had a seventy-year-old in one room and a fifty-year-old in another and could take any measure of those people, which criteria would you trust to know who was who with confidence?" Again, the answer was that only chronological age would confidently reveal the difference. Age begs for reinterpretation. Why do we conflate sickness and debility with old age? Why do we presume diminishment to our senses, sexual appetite, balance, and endurance past fifty? Who said so, and how do they know it to be true? Currently, many believe a sixty-five-year-old is too old to run for public office, too old to adopt a child, and too old to play singles in tennis. At age eighty, many are thought to be too weak to be on their own, too feeble to cook for fear of leaving the stove on, too unbalanced to ride a bicycle, and too delusional to be trusted if they think whatever ails them will get better rather than worse.

Overhearing the research participants talk amongst themselves at the beginning of the retreat made it clear that to a man they accepted these ideas and were all too aware of their "limits." They ate only the food they "knew" they could easily digest, and because they thought that their taste buds had diminished, they resisted being adventurous in their food choices. Although free to do as they pleased, they didn't even consider engaging in physical activities except those that were acceptable based on their medical histories. When John slept a little longer than he was used to and Paul was asked to do his own dishes despite his arthritis, they were initially anxious. Fred was a bit different and goaded some of the others into doing more than they were used to doing. To their surprise, everything fell into place. Instead of presuming they "couldn't" do something, they "got with the program." Where did their ideas about possibility, or more correctly impossibility, come from?

None of Us Is "Us"

Every day we learn that something we accepted as true the day before is now false. It used to be that butter was better. Then margarine was the only way to go. Now butter is back, but olive oil trumps them all. Any attempt to keep up with all the new medical findings is stressful enough that it's likely bad for our health. It's like a scene from Woody Allen's *Sleeper*, where upon awakening from a very long sleep, the protagonist discovers that everything bad is good again.

"Take that weight off or you'll be sorry." This bit of health advice is partly responsible for the diet craze omnipresent in our culture and provides some with an excuse to take dangerous drugs to help the process along. For years being overweight was seen as a psychological failure, the result of a lack of willpower. Over time, researchers began to look at the genetics of weight and found that something more might be at work—the more than fifty genes that regulate how much we eat, how active we are, and how well our bodies use calories. Then fat got even more complicated. A study showed that even twins fed quite similar diets could have very different weights. For them, at least, weight gain didn't appear to be tied to how much they ate nor the genes they inherited.

If it's not lack of will and not our genes that cause us to gain weight, maybe there's something else at work? A study of the influences of viruses on weight gain by Richard Atkinson and Nikhil Dhurandhar found that 30 percent of their obese subjects had the antibodies for a common type of adenovirus (which can cause minor illness that most of us hardly notice), while only 11 percent of the leaner subjects had them.[2] Overall, those who tested positive for the antibodies weighed significantly more than those who hadn't been infected. Further studies showed that it wasn't that fat people were more easily infected or that genetic factors were at work. Perhaps being fat in and of itself is a disease? Not so fast, say other researchers; there's no proof yet.

So, what are the facts about being overweight? Is it that we can't push back from the table soon enough, or is our desire for food programmed into us? Did we catch it, or is there something else at work? Why we gain weight, it turns out, isn't nearly as simple as most people imagine, and scientists aren't at all sure what answer to give us. It might well be that weight is due to a number of factors that differ for each one of us.

We've already touched on this kind of mindless consumption of health information in the first chapter. While it is tempting to blindly follow medical advice, it's difficult to do so when the facts keep changing. It's not science's fault; the data on which much medical advice is based are incomplete in many respects. Our bodies are complex, interconnected systems of biological processes that interact differently under the influence of the unique genetic coding and environmental factors that we each possess and experience. There is no practical way to introduce just one of these factors into a medical experiment, and no researcher would want to try. They would only face an impossible task of trying to make sense of the inordinately complicated results in looking for the causes and effects.

If we are to become good stewards of our health, we need to be certain that we have the necessary facts about it. Medical science has much to offer us. But it's not perfect, and until we appreciate the nature of how science constructs facts, we can't learn to take control of our health. We can't know everything about our health, but we can develop a mindful understanding of health through an appreciation of how medical knowledge is developed and applied. While it is tempting to mindlessly follow medical advice, it may become less so after a careful consideration of the incompleteness of the data on which the advice is based.

The instruments used to assess our health have all been created by people and thus are not perfect. The science used to assess them is probabilistic. Perhaps these diagnostic tools do predict successfully for the group, but none of us is "us."

Necessary Facts

From 1996 to 2006, the number of people seeking psychotherapy increased 150 percent, and that has put pressure on therapists and clinicians to categorize and make sense of the increased number and variety of problems in the people who seek their help. In his book *Healing Psychiatry,* Harvard psychiatrist David Brendel addresses some of the problems of applying science to mental diseases and the myth of "psychiatric scientism."[3] He notes that patients often just don't fit the diagnostic categories that clinicians use. People are too complex to fit neatly into them. The problem, as his colleague Steven Hyman describes it, is that "we have no equivalent of blood pressure cuff or blood test or brain scan that is diagnostic."[4] Indeed, scientific investigations yield probabilities that are translated by researchers, textbook writers, the media, teachers, and so on into absolute statements that are easier to talk about and teach. This leads us to think we know more than we do. Virtually all science is treated this way, with increasing simplicity.

Much of the diagnostic information on which we so readily rely when treating disease also struggles with the same simplicity-over-complexity issue: the "objective" medical measures that are used are equally suspect. Hypertension, for example, affects about fifty million Americans and is implicated in problems such as strokes, aneurysms, heart failure, heart attack, and kidney damage but can easily go unnoticed. Moreover, as physicians Sidney Port, Linda Demer, Robert Jennrich, Donald Walter, and Alan Garfinkel note in an interesting study, there is still serious debate over the exact relationship between blood pressure and mortality or even the efficacy of lowering one's blood pressure.[5] As a result, 30 percent of patients treated for hypertension may be treated inappropriately. We overlook these problems because our instruments and blood pressure charts seem so objective: a systolic reading of 140–159 indicates mild hypertension; 160–179, moderate; above 180, severe. The early stages of some of these diseases are characterized almost entirely by our measured blood pressure.

A profile of a disease may be able to tell you how to identify it, what symptoms are commonly experienced by those with it, how the disease typically progresses, and what treatment has been shown most effective for the majority of those whose experiences with the disease have been recorded, but a profile based on averages cannot tell you about our moment-to-moment experience of a condition.

Biologist Jeffrey Gordon has a fun illustration that shows how each of us can respond uniquely, in this case using a morning bowl of cereal by way of example.[6] A box of Cheerios tells us that a one-cup serving contains 110 calories. But it may be that not everyone will extract 110 calories from a cup of Cheerios. Some may extract more, some less, depending on the particular combination of microbes in their guts. "A diet has a certain amount of absolute energy," he explains. "But the amount that can be extracted from that diet may vary between individuals—not in a huge way, but if the energy balance is affected by just a few calories a day, over time that can make a big difference in body weight."

Our belief in science notwithstanding, human psychology and physiology are too complex for us to trust that the medical world is infallible. What we have to work with are correlations between observations and diseases. But the correlation is far from perfect. Scientific investigations, again, yield probabilities, not absolutes. These probabilities are translated by researchers, their textbooks, the media, teachers, parents, friends, and business managers into absolute statements that are persuasive and easy to convey. As learners, we accept what may be true under some circumstances and apply it as though it were truth across all circumstances. If instead we had been taught that something was likely in a certain context rather than definite in all, we might be less inclined to treat facts mindlessly. We would find it easier to question and rethink facts when it is in our best interest to do so.

A doctor's diagnostic tools can predict successfully across a large group of patients, but again, none of us is "us." Because findings are not absolute, subtle changes in any number of the variables that were in the original investigation could result in very big differences in the results. If we want to test a medication to see its effect on muscle strength, for example, someone has to choose the subjects, frame the information given to each participant in the study, decide what doses to test, and determine what time and under what circumstances to administer the drug. Then someone has to decide what constitutes acceptable levels of muscle strength. There are countless decisions such as these that go into every scientific study conducted. They are the "hidden decisions" that shape medical knowledge.

Again, a doctor may be able to identify a disease and describe its symptoms, how the disease typically progresses, and what treatment has been shown most effective for the majority of those whose experiences with the disease have been recorded. But she cannot predict the particular quality, location, intensity, and duration of the sensations that individuals experience, in specific parts of their body, at any given time and over time. She cannot tell you how particular individuals perceive these sensations and how closely they pay attention to them. She cannot describe what individuals are thinking or how they are coping, including their attitudes toward their condition, body, and prognosis. She cannot tell you where the individuals are or about their individual choices and behaviors at that time. In short, averages, at most, can only tell you what people tend to report experiencing and what tests tend to identify, but they do not tell you about the person.

Diagnoses, prognoses, research methods, and statistics are all necessary for efficient, ethical, and meaningful medical care, but in light of the inherent uncertainty due to variability, medicine, like all domains of study, should be regarded not as a collection of answers but rather as a way of asking questions.

Finding the questions to ask is not easy, because the facts keep changing. While exercise is surely good for us, a very recent study by Fiona Chionh, a medical oncologist, found that women who exercised a great deal were more likely to develop ovarian cancer.[7]

Exercise is good and yet exercise may be bad. Facts change. Information doesn't stand still, and this is not the fault of medical science but a reality for science in general. Let's consider the complexity of the issues involved in understanding the body. Any part of the body may affect any other part due to multiple genetic and environmental issues. An unusual allergy to pistachio nuts, insects, cleaning supplies, certain flowers, et cetera could have an effect on us. A slight imbalance in our shoes, the backpack we carry, or a reach behind a couch for the pen we dropped could do the same. Every day there are mundane experiences that put us in contact with things that could cause us problems, problems that for some of us—due to genetic vulnerability, for instance— could throw us over the proverbial edge. There is no way to factor all of this into any experiment.

A Limited Relationship: Correlation

While statistical concepts are not everyone's cup of tea, we need to take a moment to understand and appreciate the effects of two important concepts—correlation and regression—with regard to our health. Every statistics book ever written contains the phrase "correlation is not causation." It's actually a simple concept: A correlation between two pieces of information means that they are related. If the correlation in the measurement of two phenomena is positive, when the measure of one goes up, so too does the other. If the correlation is negative, their measures move in opposite directions. This does not mean that one is causing the other, however. A frequent need to urinate is correlated with diabetes, but needing to use the bathroom many times a day does not cause diabetes (nor does it mean you already have it). Correlations are rarely if ever perfect. If the correlation is statistically significant, most of the time the two factors are predictably related. What that also means is that sometimes they are not related and one factor cannot predict the other.

Not appreciating the difference between correlation and cause can have real effects. If we have a tumor, and if tumors are correlated with premature death, it cannot be said that our tumor will bring about our death. To be able to draw that conclusion, we'd have to conduct a scientific experiment that proved causation. Because of the number of variables at play, it would be very difficult if not impossible to conduct a study in a way that isolates causation clearly. It is also the case that our expectations are very important to our health. If we expect that the tumor will necessarily lead to our death, we may give up hope, and it may be giving up hope that results in our death, not the tumor.

Recent findings show that girls who are overweight before they become teenagers are more likely to be obese and have a higher risk of heart disease as women.[8] This finding may lead some girls to eat more healthfully and exercise more. So far so good. There may also be girls who learn this but fail to lose weight, even if they try. When they cannot lose weight they may, in essence, give up in the face of the information and consign themselves to their fate. They may even eat more out of fear and frustration. Thus the indirect effect of the information can be to lead some to unhealthy behavior. The medical world is only slowly acknowledging the importance of these effects.

Psychologists have conducted insightful studies of the effects of placing animals in situations where they are helpless. Important work by Martin Seligman and others on learned helplessness, for instance, found that many animals that give up actually die prematurely.[9] Seligman and his colleagues put three groups of dogs in harnesses. The control group was simply put in the harnesses for a period of time and then released. The other two groups consisted of "yoked pairs." The first group of dogs would be intentionally subjected to an electric shock, which each dog could stop by pressing a lever. For a second group of dogs, each would receive the same amount of shock as the dogs in the first group but their levers were useless; the dogs had no control over their pain. The first group of these dogs, the ones who could turn off the shock, quickly recovered from the experience, but the other dogs learned to be helpless, exhibiting symptoms similar to chronic clinical depression.

Next, the three groups of dogs were tested in a shuttle-box apparatus, in which the dogs could escape shocks by jumping over a low partition. For the most part, this last group of dogs, who had previously "learned" that they had no control over their fate, just lay down passively and whined. They didn't even try to escape the shocks.

Similar helplessness experiments have been conducted with rats.[10] The rats were restrained until they gave up trying to free themselves and became limp, and then they were placed in ice water. Rather than swim for hours, as those in the control group did (those that had not been restrained), they died soon after entering the water. Autopsies revealed that their deaths were parasympathetic. That is, they died peacefully, simply turning themselves over to their fate.

Humans demonstrate similar effects arising from positive or negative attitudes. Seligman, Christopher Peterson, and George Vaillant reanalyzed the responses to a questionnaire given to a group of Harvard men in 1946, when they were age twenty-five.[11] From the men's statements the researchers characterized each as having either a positive or pessimistic style of explaining the events of their lives. The study tracked the health and medical histories of the men for thirty-five years, and Seligman and his colleagues found that while both groups enjoyed about the same degree of health until age forty-five, those with a pessimistic explanatory style experienced poorer health between ages forty-five and sixty.

Another interesting study looked at the Chinese cultural be-

lief in fate.[12] In examining the death records of adult Chinese
Americans, the researchers found that Chinese Americans who
had a combination of disease and birth year that Chinese astrol-
ogy and medicine consider ill-fated were more likely to die. For
example, 1937 was a fire year, and the heart is the body's organ
associated with that year. A Chinese American born in 1937 was
more likely to die of heart disease than another born in a non-fire
year. Was the relationship causal? We don't know. All we have is
an interesting and suggestive correlation.

As important, our attitudes can bring about positive effects.
Psychologist Sheldon Cohen and his colleagues did some very interesting work in this area.[13] They gave subjects questionnaires
to assess emotional style and then, with their permission, quaran-
tined them and exposed them to viruses that cause colds or flu.
They found that happy people get fewer colds and flu. Regarding attitudes, here may be one area where the elderly may be su-
perior to their younger equals. Psychologist Laura Carstensen
has found that older adults are less likely to see things negatively.[14] That should make them happier and have a positive effect on their health.

Psychologists Michael Scheier and Charles Carver found a
correlation between optimism and recovery from coronary artery bypass surgery.[15] Others have studied how attitudes affect
recovery and found that this improvement is not a function of a
patient's tendency to deny that he was ill. Those who hold optimistic beliefs actually pay greater attention to their recovery, and
in so doing they aid the recovery process and help anticipate
complications. This optimism is highly correlated with mindfulness (and also may be causally related). It is well-known that people who are very ill often somehow hold on until important
events take place and then give up afterward. Similarly, when
one member of an elderly couple dies, the surviving spouse is
more likely to die soon afterward.

The consequences of giving up are quite real. When we learn a correlational finding—say, that cancer kills—and mindlessly accept it as necessarily true, then a diagnosis of cancer may unwittingly lead us to see ourselves as victims of self-fulfilling prophecies. Perniciously, any psychologically induced death that occurs only confirms the prediction—"Cancer is indeed a killer"—as if the original correlation were true for more of us than may indeed need to be the case.

Extreme Changes: Regression

Regression is the next statistical concept that we need to understand if we're going to become mindful health learners. Regression refers to the fact that behavior, feelings, and events vary around their own mean. If I hit a wonderful serve in tennis—a noticeable event for me, because it is so unusual—my next serve will probably be less good, closer to my average serve. The same phenomenon is in play if I hit a serve that is unusually bad: the next one will probably be better. Statisticians refer to this effect as "regression to the mean."

Regression to the mean is the reason why we are inclined to think that punishment is a more effective response than reinforcement. We notice the extreme. If you compliment my excellent serve, the next one will likely regress to the mean and be worse, and I may presume it is because compliments always throw me off. If you make fun of my bad serve, the next one is likely to be better and I may think I'm reacting to your negative comments and that my improvement is caused by a response to the negative comments—"I'll show you," in other words. Of course, one complication in all this is that sometimes we actually learn. Now the question becomes, Was my next serve better because I learned something about how to serve or was it because of regression to the mean? We don't know.

Ironically, the natural process of regression to the mean often makes whatever medical remedy we try seem to work. Because he had success with it, Francis Bacon believed that warts could be healed by rubbing them with pork rinds. George Washington believed that various bodily ills could be cured by passing a pair of three-inch metal rods over his body, and virtually the entire medical profession in Colonial times believed in using leeches for bloodletting to restore health. (George Washington, unfortunately, died after nine pints of blood were drained from his body in one day to treat a throat infection.) It's easy to think of Bacon, Washington, and their doctors as unscientific, but we ourselves use the same form of reasoning all the time. Again, we only notice the extreme. I felt kind of achy a couple of days ago, but now I really feel worse than usual, so I'd better take some medicine to help me get through it. The next day I feel better, so those medicines must be wonder drugs.

Because we didn't pay much attention to our minor symptoms a few days ago, when we note the more severe symptoms and take action, we probably will feel better in the near future. Is it because our symptoms have regressed to the mean or is it the medicine we took? Sometimes the medication does the job; sometimes it gets credit erroneously. In either case, it's not easy to know which is correct.

Symptoms as Cues to Disease

While a mindful learner ought to be attentive to what her body is telling her, distinguishing between that which demands attention and that which ought to be ignored can mark the fine line between being mindful and being a hypochondriac. At what point does a sensation become a symptom? Certainly, the longer it takes to recognize a symptom, the bigger a problem it may become. And yet if every unusual feeling sent us to seek advice, we'd have no time for life. What sensations do we want to consider symptoms and who makes the final decision? After how long or at what level do I call a pain a problem? We need to look at symptoms more carefully, with regard to both how we ourselves perceive them and how the medical world treats them. It turns out that symptoms are imperfect cues to disease; the correlations between the two are not perfect.

There are two very different kinds of symptoms that we treat as one, although it might serve us better if they were decoupled. There are direct symptoms that are self-evident, such as aches, pains, and fever that we observe for ourselves, and there are indirect symptoms, including blood pressure, heart rate, cholesterol, and blood sugar, that are measured by medical tests. The former are salient, demand our attention, and may be seen as their own disorder rather than as indicative of other problems. The latter are the symptoms given to us by the medical world to monitor our condition and warn us about impending problems. We'll start with them.

Many indirect symptoms present imperfect cues to disease. Let's look at cholesterol level and its correlation to heart disease, for example. Research reveals that symptoms such as high cholesterol are related to heart disease, but not everyone with high cholesterol will have a heart attack. While the correlation between high cholesterol and heart disease is a meaningful one for many people under circumstances similar to those in the research, it may or may not be so for any of us individually.

Assume that my cholesterol is very high, which suggests that I may be heading for a heart attack or stroke if I don't lower it. That information alone is stressful—which itself is not good for my health—but I proceed on the quest to lower my cholesterol level, to the exclusion of all else. (Of course, ignoring everything else makes me more vulnerable to every other disorder that is not immediately related to my level of cholesterol.) Let's assume I take medication and lower my cholesterol. My stress about my cholesterol goes away and now I don't worry so much about heart attacks.

It's like putting in a fire alarm system. I install the system so I don't have to worry about fires. With it, I can ignore the issue; the alarm system will do the work for me. Mindless to subtle cues, I may be caught unaware when the system fails. This reliance on external "devices" can lead me to be less in tune with my environment—internal and external—such that I don't notice a whiff of smoke that I might have noticed before the system went in. When I begin to take cholesterol medication, I don't want to become less in tune with my body such that I neglect or dismiss the first signs of a heart attack.

The problem with correlational research on cholesterol level and heart disease also shows itself when we consider those of us with low levels of cholesterol. Since low cholesterol is not associated with heart problems, people with low cholesterol may believe they don't have to be concerned about heart attacks. Since the correlation between cholesterol levels and heart attacks is not perfect, some people with low cholesterol levels will have heart attacks, but this group will be caught totally by surprise. This doesn't mean we shouldn't take measures such as cholesterol and blood pressure. What it does mean is that we shouldn't mindlessly rely on them. It would be more to our advantage if they guided rather than governed our thinking. I want to be clear that I am not arguing against medical tests. I am arguing against mindless reliance on them and the mindless state that they can lead to.

We also need to be aware that the way doctors frame the information they give us can have a powerful effect on our choices.

In a wonderful discussion of breast cancer screening in his book *Calculated Risks*, Gerd Gigerenzer describes four ways the data on mammography could be sensibly presented.[16] The physician could describe the relative risk, in which case having a mammogram would reduce the risk of dying from breast cancer by 25 percent. This does not mean that 25 out of 100 lives would be saved. As he explains, if we compare 1,000 women who had a mammogram with 1,000 who didn't, and 3 in the first group died compared to 4 in the second, the decrease from 4 to 3 is 25 percent and the difference in lives saved is much smaller.

Second, the physician could present the absolute risk reduction, which in this example is 1 out of 1,000. A third way to give the information would be to state the number of women who need to be treated to save one life. Here, that would be 1,000 women. Finally, Gigerenzer suggests that we could convey the increase in life expectancy that results for women ages fifty to sixty-nine who have mammograms. Surprisingly, we increase our life expectancy on average by only twelve days. Given the first but misunderstood presentation of the information, we'd be likely to get a mammogram, but given the last one, perhaps not. Framing matters, but physicians themselves are often blind to the different ways of framing medical findings. One could argue that it can't hurt to have a mammogram, so perhaps all the doctors need to do is present the first alternative. However, among other costs is the possibility of false positives—where the mammogram erroneously suggests there is a tumor. This is not a psychologically inconsequential result for the recipient of such news.

Hidden Decisions

The medical world must make decisions every day that are based on incomplete data and subject to the hidden decisions that shape the knowledge they use and deliver to us. A doctor's job is anything but simple, and it isn't as uncomplicated as it can appear.

Let's say that we need to have a tissue biopsy that might reveal that we have a cancer. Most of us expect that the procedure is definitive and without ambiguity. We arrive at the hospital, the biopsy is performed, and the tissue is sent to the lab. We expect that it will be easily determined that we either do or do not have cancer. But cancer cells do not come with labels. Someone has to examine each cell and decide whether it is a cancer cell or not. How easy is it to call one cell cancerous and another one healthy? The pathologist and the attending physician must consider any number of important questions.

- How large a sample do I need to reach an accurate diagnosis?
- What percentage of cells needs to be seen as cancerous for the patient to be diagnosed with cancer?
- When was the sample taken and under what conditions and by whom?
- If I detect cancer, what treatment do I suggest, based on what norms, and developed by whom?
- Who decides what the best treatment is, and how would it be different if someone else were to do so?
- How much do I tell the patient?
- How negative or positive should I be?
- How confident am I of my assessment?

These are just a few of the hidden decisions that are made every day and we haven't even gotten past one step in the medical process. The difficulty continues until the last set of questions has been addressed.

No two cancers are alike, so it's important to consider what a diagnosis of cancer means. A frequent method of diagnosis of cancer is a microscopic analysis of cells, also known as cytological confirmation. Included in the analysis is a blood or bone marrow smear, or aspiration or scraping of cells. People then have to make a decision: how many abnormal cells do there have to be to indicate "cancer"? A cytology technician can examine tens of millions of cells a day in the search for malignancies. Whatever cutoff point is used to decide that someone does or does not have cancer, some people will fall just below this number.

It doesn't matter what the cutoff point is. There will always be some who fall just below that point and others just above it. A group of people with their own understanding of what is correct made the decision in the face of uncertainty—and the result for those who fall just above it can be devastating, just as those who fall just below it may become overly optimistic. Despite the fact that people in the first group may be very close to those of the second, they may face a course of treatment that is difficult and un-settling. In all cases, someone makes a decision that could affect their entire lives. It's not just our health at stake, these decisions can upturn our emotional, social, and professional lives. IQ test scores, for example, have been used as the basis for classifying people's abilities far beyond their accuracy. A score of 80 is not statistically different from a score of 79, although the label that attaches to the lower score would certainly have lasting, negative effects if it's mindlessly imposed on us.

Doctors make these decisions based on the best science possible, and it is often very good science indeed, but there are any number of hidden decisions that go into medical research. There are only so many people who can participate in a study. Those people who never find their way into the study are excluded from consideration, as are those who recover on their own.

When researchers say that the research participants were drawn at random from the general population, what does this really mean and what difference might the differences make? Harry is a multimillionaire, while Jane is struggling to find the money to feed her four young children; Arnie hasn't left the house for days for fear of having to socialize; Linda won't even answer her telephone because she's always pressed against an important deadline. The very wealthy, the very poor, the very shy, and the very busy are not as likely to be included in experiments, and that limits our knowledge about the "general" population. When our health is compared to norms, we need to ask on whom these norms were based. Norms are always more ambiguous than they seem. We have a norm for how much sleep we need, for example. Over $2.5 billion was spent on sleeping pills in 2006. It leads me to question whether the norms about how much sleep we need may be inaccurate and whether we need to ask, "Needed for what?" rather than accept that so many of us are sleep-deprived.

When a study is not based on a robust, truly random sample of the population, the data are less trustworthy. One recent study of more than seventy thousand women—a very robust sampling—shows that older women who take hormone pills that combine estrogen and testosterone more than double their risk of breast cancer.[17] All the seventy thousand women in the study also happened to be nurses, which qualifies the robustness of the sample—an increased risk of breast cancer may be specific to nurses rather than the general population. Are those women who choose to become nurses more similar to one another than to the general population of women? And if so, is this similarity an important risk factor? We simply don't know, which is why scientific research is an almost constant search for better truths and not "the truth." We can ask whether a sample is ever really truly random, such that pygmies and professors are equally likely to be represented.

Subject selection is just the beginning of the set of decisions that go into the social construction of our health. At each stage of the medical process, from diagnosis to treatment, something must be left out, leaving much room for error. Disease aside, the same questions of who is deciding, based on what criteria, and how things would be different if someone else made the decision come into play in regard to notions of all aspects of health and well-being. Mix together cultural norms and patient attitudes, and suddenly the limitations of medical research and our health, in the broad sense of how we as individuals actually experience our lives, are as much a matter of "says who?" as of expert science.

Becca Levy and I conducted a study to explore whether cultural attitudes and stereotypes about old age might contribute to physical decline that is associated with growing older, in this case memory loss. We wanted to compare the stereotypes many of us hold with the attitudes of people who generally don't have negative stereotypes about old age. In order to look at people who weren't burdened by such stereotypes, in addition to a random sampling of young people and adults with normal hearing, we recruited young and elderly members of two communities—the mainland Chinese (where elders are held in high esteem) and deaf Americans (who don't generally share the hearing world's negative views of old age). We gave each group a questionnaire that asked, "What are the first five words or descriptions that come to mind when you think of someone old?" As expected, the Chinese and the deaf were less likely to mention memory loss than the other groups. The research question for us was whether this absence of a negative stereotype for memory loss would lead to better memory for the elders in these groups than for mainstream U.S. culture. Or, to put this another way, we hypothesized that negative stereotypes about memory adversely affect memory.

Because these two populations have so little in common other than their regard for the elderly, we reasoned that similar responses on memory tests would give weight to our view. Our hypothesis was that if negative views contribute to memory loss in old age, and the Chinese people and deaf Americans hold more positive views of aging than Americans who have their hearing, mainland Chinese and deaf Americans should show less memory loss with aging. We compared the performance of mainland Chinese and deaf Americans in memory tests and found that while younger people from the groups all performed equally well, the older mainland Chinese and older deaf Americans tested better than older hearing Americans. If memory loss in old age was determined primarily by biology, older subjects would be expected to demonstrate the same memory skills.

The results seem to indicate that age-related changes in our health do not inevitably mean decline. Research on memory loss in general bears out this conclusion. Though some researchers have argued that such a decline is inevitable and have documented consistent trends to that effect, others believe that some aspects of the deterioration of memory may be environmentally determined, shaped by expectations and social contexts. Admittedly, as with all research, we made decisions as to the parameters of the study: for example, of all possible subcultures in the world, we chose two based on our understanding of their lack of bias in this area.

Mindless Labels and Mindful Decisions

Whatever our condition, the cues in our environment that prime our symptoms and the symptoms themselves change from day to day and even hour to hour. The question we face is to decide which symptoms are the "real" ones and which are socially constructed. Should we simply let others decide no matter what the consequences?

Consider the direct symptom of "chronic pain." How often does something have to hurt before the pain is considered chronic? Once a day for ten minutes? An hour? Every other day?

How intense does the pain have to be? Who decided? How did they make this decision? The decision is not trivial. Once our pain is labeled "chronic" we expect it to occur and we overlook instances of its nonoccurrence. It is in these nonoccurrences that our control lies.

We experience symptoms directly or indirectly, and if the symptoms are intense enough, the medical world then tries to find a label for them. It is easy to see the advantages of symptom labeling; after all, it helps us create a common experience. If I have stomach pains, go to the doctor, and am diagnosed with gastroenteritis, several things result. First, I feel validated that the pain is real and not psychosomatic. I can also more easily talk to people about my disorder, and with a name comes the belief that I am not alone in this experience. With the belief that others have this condition comes the belief that relief, if not immediately available, may soon be found. Finally, there is a benefit for the medical world—different groups of researchers can more easily all study the same problem, possibly finding a treatment more quickly.

The disadvantages of symptom labeling are more subtle. Most important among these subtleties is the way labels lead us to give up control. This happens in several ways: Labeling promotes excessive dependence on experts and technology. It also leads us to compartmentalize ourselves, such that health cues from other parts of our bodies are more likely now to be neglected. A label leads us to accept as stable something that in fact is ever variable. Once we as individuals or a culture believe we know what something is, we are less likely to look at it anew.

Labels lead us to draw distinctions between what fits and what doesn't. For instance, the medical world has given us two labels for our symptoms: "real" and "psychosomatic." The distinction itself promotes reliance on the expertise of others once we accept it, even though to us, we feel the same in both cases. The distinction, while perhaps useful in some ways to some people, is still potentially harmful. In one sense, all disorders are psychosomatic; all pain is psychological.

The diagnosis that a condition is "psychosomatic" means that medical science believes it cannot help us. It does not mean the pain is not real. But because persistent pain often engages us in a battle to show "them" (doctor after doctor) that it is real, we give up our control. In fact, if we notice when the pain diminishes, we might figure out how to control it when it is present or just let it continue diminishing.

Many disorders that now have "respectable" names were at one time deemed to be psychosomatic—and the person with the disorder often considered a hypochondriac. Before we had an understanding of arthritis, someone who complained about pain in her fingers, pain in her neck, and pain in her knees might have qualified as a hypochondriac. The first thing, then, to note about hypochondriacs is that the future may give a name to their symptoms and thus free them from that pejorative label. Second, there may be clues in their symptoms that, if taken seriously, could reveal something systemic. If, for example, we kept track of the things people complained of and found that certain symptoms appear together, we might discover a new disorder or a new way of looking at an existing one. Thus, several of the disorders that are seen as psychosomatic today may be labeled as "true" diseases tomorrow.

Few, if any, would dispute the fact that our psychology plays a part in our reaction to and the course of our diseases. The only question is how large a part. The answer is that we cannot really know. If we assume it is a large part, the perceived possibility of controlling our bodies increases exponentially.

How would things be different if we viewed all disease as psychosomatic? If this were the case, it might seem unreasonable and perhaps irresponsible not to try to heal ourselves. We have mistakenly been convinced that our bodies are separate from our minds. Many of us admit that we don't know much about our biology. Few of us, however, believe that we have no control over our minds.

Whether or not it is important that we label disease, we need to ask who does the labeling. Consider erectile dysfunction and those responsible for deciding whether this is a disorder for which medication should be prescribed, and thus whether insurance companies must pay the bill. If the decision makers at the insurance companies were all women, we might get a very different result than if the deciders were a group of lusty men of the same age. The women might also be more likely to suggest that insurance companies cover birth control pills. Whenever there is a decision to be made, there are decision makers who have values and motivations that may or may not coincide with our own. When disease is considered in this light, we may have more motivation to enter into our own care.

When there is a decision to be made, that means there is uncertainty. When there is uncertainty, there are choices about how much information to consider, what information is relevant, and what is not. There are decisions to be made about what to consider a cost and what to consider a benefit. At each decision point, values enter the equation. Even if that were not the case, although it necessarily is, the scientific data that are being considered are probabilistic, not absolute, suggesting still more uncertainty. If we don't embrace that uncertainty, the decisions are made for us, the uncertainty is hidden from view, and the rest unfolds according to traditional practice, leaving us with few or no alternatives.

Healthy or Ill?

When the results of our biopsy bring us a diagnosis of cancer, a profound change often happens. Many of us lose our earlier identities and become a "cancer patient," a label that opens us up to all the negative effects of labels. But that needn't be the case. Recent work by psychologist Sarit Golub has shown that we have a choice about how we accept and apply those labels.[18] Her work found that some people add cancer to their identity, so to speak, while others let the diagnosis take over their identity. The former group fares better on most measures of recovery and psychological well-being.

An interesting aspect of her work is how patients' ratings of their quality of life don't always agree with their physicians' assessment of their physical health. Her research suggests that the largest factor in determining quality of life is the way that people think about the relationship between their identity and their illness. People who felt damaged by their illness tended to rate their quality of life as low, while others who saw the limitations imposed by the disease as an opportunity for growth tended to rate their quality of life as higher. Golub cites Lance Armstrong's declaration that "cancer is literally the best thing that ever happened to me" as a high-profile example.

If we compared people who fall just short of a diagnosis with those who are just at or above the cutoff, and followed both groups over time, what would we find? I think they would become less and less alike. One group may become healthy while the other remains cancer patients—even though the original difference between them and another diagnosis was not meaningfully different statistically.[19] What differs is our reaction to the diagnosis.

A disease presents itself as a set of symptoms. Those who have these symptoms, do nothing, and are fine are not part of the analysis—they never present themselves to the medical world. Thus it is impossible to know how strong the relationship is between these symptoms and subsequent health effects. Moreover, the self-fulfilling aspects of calling these symptoms a disease is unknown. Yet lives would be meaningfully different based on test results that are not meaningfully different.

We look at ourselves and declare that we are either healthy or sick. Despite the tendency to sort people into just two categories, probably no one would argue against the idea that health exists on a continuum. Not only do people vary from person to person in "how much" of an illness they have, they also vary in how intense the illness is for them at any particular time. When my arms and legs are strong and I can breathe like an Olympic swimmer and I have an infection in my ear, am I healthy or sick? When my vision and hearing are excellent and my lungs are strong and I have MS, am I healthy or sick? If our beliefs were inconsequential to our health, it would make no difference, but here the argument is that our beliefs are crucial to our well-being.

Andre Dubus, the wonderful short-story writer, was in a horrible accident that left his legs paralyzed. In his book *Meditations from a Movable Chair*, he offers a vivid illustration of the choice we have available to us.

> "You were hit by a silver—" She named a car I know nothing about, but not the right one.
> I said: "It was a Honda Prelude."
> "And it paralyzed you?"
> "No. Only my legs are useless. I'm very lucky. I had three broken vertebrae in my back. But my spine was okay. My brain."

Consider what life would be like if we gave up the idea of healthy or sick—zero versus one—and replaced it with the idea of multiple continua. One minute, for example, we might score 60 percent on one health dimension, 30 percent on another, and perhaps 85 percent on yet a third. How would that change our lived experience? First, we could still feel empowered because we would recognize that much of our body is still working just fine. Second, it is easier to try to "fix" a smaller problem (60 percent healthy) than a big one (100 percent sick). Third, we would have many more people to whom we might compare ourselves and thereby potentially find many more solutions to our health. If you have only 30 percent of the problem and have found a solution, maybe it could work for me at 60 percent. That's a lot easier to imagine than in the all-or-none world in which we currently find ourselves.

Of course, no doctor, no matter how close to us, no matter how earnest and caring he or she might be, is going to do all those calculations. Once we start to do it for ourselves, we're sure to run into the problem of how and when we figure it all out. Just how bad is my particular disease, given how good these other parts of me are? As we collect the data on ourselves, we should notice that we keep changing on each continuum. All of this should be a very mindful activity, leading to even more attention to variability. At some point as we become very sophisticated with the process, we should notice similarities and differences over time and that what affects one issue may also affect another. For example, the exercises I've been doing to improve my back have also affected my balance and the pain in my foot. If I come to see that using my nondominant hand for some tasks helps my posture, which helps my back pain, I even may find that my hearing has improved, although the link right now is not straightforward. Eventually—only eventually—we may get to a place where we don't need the continua; we may one day be in a place where we spontaneously notice subtle signals our bodies give and make the necessary corrections as part of our ongoing lived experience.

My friend Elaine tells the story of friends of hers, a female couple, one of whom was a doctor. The nondoctor experienced chest pains while driving and immediately called her doctor partner. Knowing her very well and having little reason based on the science she had learned in medical school to believe her significant other was a likely candidate for a heart attack, the doctor said she was probably having indigestion. Doctor or no doctor, the woman in pain was scared and accordingly drove herself to the hospital anyway. It turned out to be a heart attack.

CHAPTER 5

Reengineering Medical Rules

The only man I know who behaves sensibly is my tailor; he takes my measurements anew each time he sees me. The rest go on with their old measurements and expect me to fit them.

—George Bernard Shaw

Imagine a situation in which an elderly woman is able to live independently. She typically shops for her groceries every few days. When she arrives at her apartment door, she puts down the grocery bag, searches for her key, opens the door, and then bends down to pick up the bag and carries it inside. Today, however, is different. She puts the bag down but can't bend over far enough to pick it up. Luckily, a neighbor happens by to help her, but the problem persists. If she can't get her groceries home, she is no longer able to take care of herself. Her adult children, fearing for her diminished state, help her move to a nursing home.

Now consider this scenario. An elderly woman living independently comes back to her apartment with her groceries. She places the bag on a small shelf outside her door, searches for her key, opens the door, and carries in her grocery bag. In the first case, the woman is considered too frail to care for herself, but not in the latter. The only difference is a small piece of wood serving as a shelf.

The external world is socially constructed, but we rarely see it that way. Most things were initially designed to meet the needs of the designer and that person's conception of the "typical" person. The width of a seat in a theater, the height of a kitchen table, and the size of a sugar cube were all decisions that might not best meet our individual needs. The problem is that we often don't see much of our external world. It's in the background, unchanging and unchallenged, blinding us to the fact that choices were made in its construction. If our socially constructed environment ceases to work for us, we see it as a fault of ours. It rarely occurs to us to attribute the problem to the environment or to change the construction to meet our needs. When I reach for a dish on the top shelf in the kitchen and accidentally drop it, I may attribute the broken plate to my clumsiness. It would be better for me to forget the personal insult and attribute it to being distracted as I reached for the plate. It would be even better, however, to recognize that the shelf was built for someone taller than I am. Perhaps with this realization, I might even decide to have the shelves redesigned to better fit *my* needs.

The shape of the medical world affects our views of ourselves and our health and it too is socially constructed. Doctors and nurses wear uniforms, hospital rooms are all similar, bandages are white, IV poles are ominous-looking, doctors' offices are bar-

ren except for framed degrees, patients doors are left open—
most everything about the medical world as it is constructed is a
double-edged sword, although we rarely recognize the negative
effects or challenge their reason for being.

Let's take these up in turn. Medical uniforms serve certain important functions: they denote group affiliation, and they are
white so that dirt and other contaminants can be easily spotted.
Medical uniforms also confer status on the wearer. Each of these
functions comes at a cost, which varies depending on the context.
If we visit a doctor in her office, do we need to see her in a white
coat to know that she is our doctor? The uniform creates distance
and implicitly keeps us in our place. It tells us who the expert is
here, and so we are less likely to question her, even if questioning would be to our advantage. If the doctor needed to perform
some messy procedure, at that time a lab coat could be donned. In
a nursing home setting, elderly adults are not likely to be confused with staff; the latter probably don't need to wear uniforms.
When they do, they emphasize "nursing" over "home." Whatever the advantages of uniforms, their disadvantages bear thinking about.

What is the effect of the uniform on the wearer? Deciding
what to wear every day presents the opportunity to examine how
we are feeling psychologically (and physically)—if only we were
to ask why we make the choices we do. This information could
be useful. By choosing our clothes, we become more individualized, and that could lead us to take more responsibility for our actions. While our uniforms convey status, it is easy for us to hide
behind status. Years ago, when consulting to a nursing home,
I vividly remember how dramatically my experience changed
when I first thought about uniforms. I didn't have a uniform
proper, but I walked around with a pen and pad on which I rarely
wrote anything down. They were my uniform, and I found that
I hid behind them. My "uniform" announced that I was a person

of status. It determined how the staff would view and interact with me and how I in turn would interact with them. I didn't need to fully engage. After all, I was in charge. On my third visit to one of these homes, I decided to put the pad and pen away. Going without my "uniform" forced me be in the present as a person, not as someone with a particular status earned in the past. I found it exhilarating and I began to look forward to my time at that facility, which I used to dread.

I soon suggested that the nurses put their uniforms away as well. They at first strenuously objected but in the end followed suit. I was consulting to the nursing home and not doing research, so I didn't collect data, but once the uniforms were put away, the difference in the nursing home was almost palpable. Individuals interacted with other individuals. While there were still differences among residents, nurses, doctors, and consultant, especially age-related ones, these differences—and the status associated with the roles—became less a factor in dealing with everyday problems. Residents seemed to be less demanding of the nurses, and nurses seemed to be more respectful of the residents.

Why should the everyday external world have such negative effects on the very people that the medical establishment is trying to help? Perhaps the answer can be found in the growing body of social psychological research on how past experience influences our current behavior in ways that we are often unaware of. It often takes very little to make such experiences salient.

Psychologists Anthony Greenwald and Mahzarin Banaji refer to the cues that activate particular associations and influence our behavior as "primes."[1] Our physical environment primes our feelings and behavior, although we are typically oblivious to its influence. Primes often tell us what is expected of us, and too often we mindlessly comply. Many aspects of the medical world do just this in ways that are not helpful, presenting us with subtle cues that lead us to behave in ways we otherwise would not behave. In a sense they control our behavior. Psychologists John Bargh, Mark Chen, and Lara Burrows conducted a wonderful study to understand more deeply the effects of priming and to consider its potential negative effects.[2] Subjects were randomly put into one of two groups. In the experimental group, they were asked to solve anagrams, unaware that they had been formed from words that were stereotypes about old age (for example, *felorguft* from *forgetful*). The control group solved anagrams of neutral, non-age-related words. After solving the anagrams, people were purportedly finished with their participation and dismissed. The researchers then timed their short walk to the elevator in order to leave the building. Those research participants whose anagrams contained primes for "old age" walked to the elevator more slowly.

In more recent work, my students Maja Djikic and Sarah Stapleton and I were interested in seeing if we could reverse the effects of mindless primes.[3] Before we started the study proper we had people sort a hundred photographs of old and young individuals. We found that if young people sort mixed photos of old and young people, the photos prime old age. In our experiment, those in the control group were instructed to put the photos into two groups, "old" or "young," twenty at a time, thus priming them for old age. This group replicated the slowed walking speed of the previous study's subjects. An experimental group sorted the photos into several groups where, for each twenty photos, they were given a new, non-age-related category (such as "gender") on which to base the sorting. A second experimental group generated their own non-age-related sorting categories. We were looking to see whether the mindful action of recategorizing would lead people to be immune to the "old age" prime. We expected them to come to see the person in the photo was many things and not just old. The experimental groups that did the mindful sorting did not walk slowly. Being mindful allowed them to overcome the effects of the "old age" prime.

The Socially Constructed World

White coats in hospitals may work the same way. They prime the concept "doctor" and so they bring to mind our stereotypes about doctors. If we see doctors as authority figures instead of as people first, we tend to behave as though they are just that, even if a particular doctor may be very approachable. Doctor and nurse uniforms are also likely to prime "patient" as well, and when we see ourselves as patients, we tend to behave like them.

Most doctors' offices are rather sterile and uninviting, conveying to patients the seriousness of their visit, even when it may not be very serious. Almost every aspect of a hospital room suggests serious illness. Not only does this affect the patient directly by inducing stress, but it affects him indirectly through his family and friends. Imagine you come to see me in the hospital and you see that I'm on an IV. Where would you stand and how do you interact with me? Now imagine that the pole from which the IV hangs is playfully candy-striped, like a child's image of the North Pole. Where might you stand and how do you interact with me? (Of course, if the pole has always been striped, we might associate candy striping with ominous needles. The larger point is that often we are oblivious to the effect of the environment on our behavior.)

Imagine that you are recovering from knee surgery after an early winter ski accident. When you're ready to get up and around on your crutches, you might realize that whoever made them didn't think that winter ambulation was a good idea. If crutches were made so that you could press a button to release metal cleats, you would not necessarily be so house-bound.

In nursing homes, life is made as easy as possible for the residents. On the face of it, this seems to be a good thing. Without any difficulties, however, there is little room for any feeling of mastery. If we truly wanted life to be easy, we would make very different choices than most of us currently do. We would only ski on beginners' slopes; we'd be content to play just scales on our musical instruments; we'd rarely if ever try anything new. Clearly, most of us want to be challenged intellectually, physically, or both. To master something new feels good and fosters mindfulness, which is good for us and our health. And there is more benefit to the process of actively mastering (because it is mindful) than having already mastered. The elderly are often deprived of these advantages. Not only do we make life too easy for them, but we overassist them with whatever difficulties we can't completely eliminate. Helping feels good to the helper, but over time it may make the helped feel incompetent. Dr. Jerry Avorn of Harvard Medical School and I conducted research in which we either guided elderly adults in a task, directly helped them, or let them fend for themselves.[4] The results were clear: those who were helped performed the most poorly at the task. I'm not suggesting that we stop being helpful. I am suggesting that we think twice in each instance and ask if, given a bit more time, the person could help herself. If she does, she helps herself to be healthier.

Another group we overhelp is the "disabled." Handicapped signs label us as such and suggest that our abilities are steady-state. There are days any of us can walk a good distance and days that it is harder, but how often do I ask myself what I feel I can do today if I have a handicapped parking sticker and always make use of the allotted spaces? The way to deal with infirmity is not to ignore it or hide it; rather, the world we construct could and should do a better job of conveying to us that our abilities vary from day to day and that the disorders we have are not fixed. (Some parking lots have a minibus that drives around, picking up anyone who wants a ride, eliminating the need to sequester those with a need for help to a specific area of the lot.) Some of the changes that could be made don't require much work, just new thinking. Consider one of my pet peeves: open-door policies in nursing homes and hospitals. The open door not only deprives us of privacy but also implicitly tells us we are weak and in need of constant supervision. While an open door may be useful on a critical care ward, the human costs may be unnecessarily high for others. Anything that subtly tells us we need total care fosters dependency, passivity, and mindlessness. When we are encouraged to depend so completely on others, we don't need to pay attention to how we may be able to care for ourselves today. If we were brought into the process of caring for ourselves, we probably would think to pay attention to subtle changes in our health, to take charge of at least some of the things we can do ourselves, and in so doing improve our psychological and physical state.

Medical equipment shouts that we are sick. Does the grab bar in the shower have to look so categorically out of place? It could be designed to fit more discreetly into the overall design. Can't crutches be more aesthetically appealing? When I was a graduate student, I saw someone wearing a cast that was colorfully painted. It invited the observer to look, indeed to stare at the person's misfortune. It occurred to me that at least part of the reason we avoid people with handicaps is because they create a conflict for us. We're curious and want to look, but we're not supposed to stare.

Colleagues Shelley Taylor, Susan Fiske, Benzion Chanowitz, and I decided to test this psychological conflict between wanting to stare and the desire to follow our social norms against staring, what we called the novel-stimulus hypothesis.[5] We wanted to see if when people were given the chance to satisfy their curiosity, they would be less likely to avoid disabled people when they encountered them.

We conducted experiments in which student participants were allowed to observe a person with a large leg brace through a one-way mirror, and then measured how close the student sat to the person when later in the same room. Not surprisingly, we found that those students who were allowed to stare sat closer than those who were suddenly introduced to the person and asked to sit with him or her.

The FAA has a checklist for airline pilots to use as a safety check. The checklist is now so familiar that many pilots run through it mindlessly, which has resulted in an increase in accidents. Likewise, one of the most damaging artifacts of our socially constructed medical world is the medical chart. First, these charts don't change much, and in this regard, the medical staff, just like the pilots, may learn to treat them mindlessly. The categorical information that is the focus of these charts—information such as past medical history, psychological history, medications, allergies—is based on what is necessary for the typical patient. Idiosyncratic information that might be important can get lost. Research reveals new findings every day, but charts are upgraded infrequently. Consider if instead we redesigned these charts so that they required the doctor to look intently at the patient (perhaps to gauge pallor or alertness or temperament) in order to complete part of them; the information gathered and tallied would by necessity be different each time the doctor or nurse used the chart. Now the doctor would have to actively engage the patient, and the patient would feel individualized and engage the doctor. The interaction would go from mindless to mindful, and the health and well-being of both patient and doctor would improve.[6]

The technology already exists to make the environment (both the general environment and the medical environment) more accommodating to an older population. For example, older people often find cell phones, PDAs, and the like hard to read because the screen fonts were created by and for young people. As long as our culture teaches us that vision must get worse as we age, there is a ready market awaiting the person who redesigns these devices for those of us with less acute vision and a lack of desire to find out how to program the larger font. In the same way, medication typically used to be tested on young adults. As a result, older adults were often overmedicated. If the reverse had been the case, younger adults would seem beyond treatment—the drugs just would not have been as effective. Some of us who are young resemble the old, and just as certainly some of us who are old resemble the young; thus some of us are not getting enough medication and some are getting too much.

What if, instead of writing a prescription for a single medication, the doctor gave us a choice of at least two medications that she believed would be beneficial? That would not only bring us into the process and increase our mindfulness but also remind the physician of the uncertainty inherent in the choice in the first place. It might even be enough to lead us to stay tuned in over time while we take the chosen medication, revealing the variability in our symptoms to us.

In changing our houses and offices—all aspects of the environment—so that there is a better fit for us, we might be surprised by improvements in health that could follow. But why end there? Perhaps there is a way to prevent some of the diminished capacities that accompany aging. What if we created virtual aging and virtual disease to enable people when younger and healthy to learn how better to cope with and overcome many of the symptoms they may eventually experience? Let's go back to the assumption that as we age, our field of vision narrows and we become more sensitive to cold. A thirty-degree day feels different in February than it does in October, regardless of the sweaters we may wear. While we adapt to seasonal changes, we typically don't adjust to age-related changes. If younger people, say in their forties or fifties, were exposed to a narrowing field of vision and increased sensitivity to cold, we could learn how to deal with these and other age-related changes while still feeling strong. Because the situation would be novel for us as younger adults, increased attention to variability in our reactions (a mindful response) could very well follow. With attention to variability comes an increase in perceived control, which in turn will make us pay more attention to the situation; an increase in mindfulness will increase health and increase our control over the symptoms. Having learned how to "deal with" age-related changes, we would be better fit to face our own aging. If we assume problems are a necessary consequence of aging about which we can do nothing, on the other hand, we do not expend the time or energy looking for ways to decrease or reverse them.

Sometimes the solution is right at hand, like the shelf described above, and we do not need to create virtual worlds. My grandmother would turn the thermostat up. My mother would turn it down. Each thought the other abnormally cold or hot, respectively, but since they both accepted that old people are generally the ones with the "problems," my grandmother most often lost the battle of the thermostat. If they had not looked at differences in this way, they might have easily solved the problem by respectively putting on or taking off a sweater before having an argument about it.

Another reason why we need to attend to the fit between ourselves and our environments is because of the way we still mindlessly process environments when we are young adults. Often when we furnish our houses, we buy a table, a couch, some chairs, and a bed, for example. After we've lived with them for a short while, we cease to notice them, if we ever really did. We're often too busy to devote much time to the subtleties of the items around us. If when we are older we are confined more or less to our houses, it won't now occur to us to see these things in new ways. That is, initially we mindlessly learn to ignore our physical world because we are too busy. Then later, when we are unnecessarily left with too little to think about, it doesn't occur to us to think about anything we've mindlessly previously understood. That doesn't mean we have to mindfully engage everything even if we could. The alternative is simply not to learn about it mindlessly at the beginning, so in the future it could occur to us to think about it anew. For example, rarely do older adults think to change their rooms around to meet their current needs. The furniture stays put for life, and discarding the table they no longer use, for instance, never comes up for consideration.

Many of us have accepted that we have problems when in fact what may be going on is a poor fit between our lifestyle or occupation and the "problem." For example, if a job required shifting among many things, ADHD might not be a problem. On the other hand, if we were very energetic, it would be hard to collect tolls all day. Before we conclude that we don't fit into the world, it would behoove us to consider where we might fit better.

The Importance of Roles

I once slipped on a sheet of ice and found myself in the hospital for the next two weeks, recuperating from a smashed ankle. There I was a patient, a participant, an observer, and, when the pain passed, a psychologist. It was a very revealing two weeks.

It was six-thirty in the morning. I had already been in the hospital for several days, but this was the first one where the drugs I had been given didn't affect my memory. A nurse came in the room and announced that she was going to take my vital signs. I said only one word to her: "Hi." She immediately changed her demeanor, exclaiming that I was a breath of fresh air and had made her day. At first I was startled that such a small gesture of recognition on my part had such a big effect. Then I talked to her about it. She told me, not surprisingly, that people don't like to be awakened and that most of the time they are very unpleasant when she had to do so. In these instances, patients treat nurses as the enemy. Nurses expect this and often preemptively act their part in the drama. In these situations, there are no people present, just patients and nurses, each enacting their role. Add a person and the drama changes for the better for both parties.

Another time, I rang the bell for help and a nurse entered and asked what I needed. As I began to tell her why I had rung, I realized that she was weighing my need against her availability, and this is most often the case. If a nurse is busy, she will find my request burdensome and she will resent the request. Patients, however, cannot know how busy the nurses are at any particular time. We ring the bell and wait, and eventually someone comes. If it takes awhile, the patient feels ignored and nurses feel put upon. Imagine instead that people took the place of nurses and patients.

Patient rings bell. Nurse enters.

PATIENT: "Hi, is it busy right now?"

NURSE: "Yes. Several nurses had to go to the second floor for some emergency. What do you need?"

PATIENT: "Can someone come help me get to the chair when they have a moment?"

NURSE: "Sure. It may be a few minutes, though."

It's going to take as long as it takes in any case. Now, however, the wait is met with understanding rather than mounting hostility. Or take the more difficult request for a bedpan to be removed. No one wants to do it, nor should they, but it must be done. If it is done in role, there is often resentment on the part of the aide and perhaps guilt or feelings of helplessness on the patient's part. I said to a nurse in this circumstance, "I'm sorry, I wish I had another option." She felt bad and said, "Don't think twice about it; it's part of my job." She no longer resented my request, and I felt grateful rather than guilty.

One morning, the occupational therapist arrived and announced, "I am the OT. My name is Jane." I replied, "Hello, I'm Ellen. What did you say your name was?" "I'm Jane." By separating her name from her rank and serial number, she seemed more a person to me. The ensuing session was person to person. This is important because much of the advice medical people are trained to give is really one size fits all, and so to adjust it to our individual needs we need to feel free to ask questions, to refuse some of what we are offered in the way of help, or to ask for more if we need it. I wanted to do upper-body exercises while I waited for my ankle to heal. It wasn't part of the program, and it would have been hard to ask the OT or PT to help me. It was much easier asking Jane.

Psychologist Adam Grant and I decided to put this idea to the test.[7] Subjects were presented with a scenario and asked what they would do in that situation. Half of the people were presented with the following situation: You're in the hospital, on a bedpan, and very uncomfortable. Your usual nurse is unavailable. There is another nurse outside your room. How likely are you to ask her for help? The other half of the participants were given this scenario: You're in the hospital, on a bedpan, and very uncomfortable. Your usual nurse, Betty Johnson, is unavailable. There is another nurse outside your room. How likely are you to ask her for help? The only difference between the two groups is whether or not their usual nurse is named. Naming one nurse seems to have suggested that perhaps all nurses are people as well as nurses and that they could be approached more easily than nameless nurses. We found that when roles were replaced with a name, more people replied that they would ask for help.

There is an even more important reason to "pass the role" whenever we can, and that is that mistakes arise from mindlessness. If our interactions with others are not individual in nature, they risk unfolding in a mindless manner. Role-to-role behavior is rule-bound and normative; that is, a typical pattern of behavior is likely to be repeated. There are times when the rules should not be followed, but to notice these instances requires that we pay attention to the way this situation is different. This can be hard for medical staff, because they always see so many patients and tend not to distinguish among them, although it would be to their advantage. But it should not be hard for patients, because we typically are not always patients and we have fewer people to keep track of. And as with the staff, it is clearly in our best interest to do so. It is easier for us to stay mindful if we are who we are and not what our patient role may "demand."

Once a nurse wanted to take blood to test my sugar level. I am not a diabetic person, and I politely questioned the need for the test. As a patient, I might not have. The nurse then realized that she had the wrong person/patient, and I assume she moved along to find the right one.

CHAPTER 6

Words in Context

Words differently arranged have a different meaning and meanings differently arranged have a different effect.

—Blaise Pascal

We all know that good communication fosters healthy relationships. When two people "speak the same language," they both presume they see the same world and share common experiences. We use language to communicate essential facts about the world and our experience in it. For the most part, it serves us well. Language does, however, lead us to believe we know less than we could; it often creates a naive realism and an illusion of knowing that comes with many built-in limitations.

When we all use the same words, we can easily get lulled into thinking we are having the same experience, when in fact our experiences may be very different. One way to look at it is that our experience is in motion, but our language holds that experience still. Our description of last night's Red Sox game—"It was a close game, but in the bottom of the ninth inning the batter hit a walk-off home run"—while informative, doesn't capture our felt experience.

Language needn't be explicitly verbal; cues are so often paired with language that we are able to understand other people by their nonverbal behavior alone. Take a simple sound, for example, "psst." Using only that sound, try having a conversation with someone where you want to communicate anger. "Psst, psst, psst"—your tone can tell another person how you feel. Now try to communicate appreciation and caring. It works just as well here. Language writ large—verbal and nonverbal together—is a highly social activity that leads us to ignore individual experience and seek to engage that which is common among us, and so we learn to listen to the outside world instead of listening to ourselves. When you ask me how I feel and I tell you I have a stomachache, I presume that your experience of stomachaches enables you to understand that I feel reasonably unwell. But the many possible differences between our experiences get lost, as language creates an illusion of knowing. Language is shorthand; individual experience is the full text.

I recently visited a dentist who told me at one point in the procedure that I would feel pressure. I didn't feel pressure and I didn't feel any pain. I did not know how to describe what I did feel and so I said nothing. In truth, I ignored the experience, because it didn't fit the language of the situation. It might not have mattered at the time, but any information I don't convey might be very important in different situations, so there may be an advantage in coming to better know our individual experience. At the least, I probably should have said that I was having difficulty describing what I was experiencing. At that point, I hope, he'd ask me questions that helped me to convey it.

Language too often binds us to a single perspective. By dint of their experience and training, doctors and patients come to the table speaking and hearing different languages. What the doctor understands when I say "It hurts a bit" may be quite different from what I mean to communicate. I might be trying to tolerate what is in fact a good deal of pain, and she hears that the pain is not a big problem. I might also be feeling very little pain, but she hears that I have a pain worthy of intervention and medication. We don't often question information when it comes to us from an authority or it is presented in absolute and unyielding language. We simply accept it and become trapped in a fixed mindset, oblivious to the fact that authorities are sometimes wrong or overstate their case, or that language can be highly manipulative. When doctors speak with us, we all too often take their insights as revelations and their advice as dictum.

Imagine an approach that opens us up to uncertainty, which opens us up to possibility. If doctors simply preceded statements with phrases such as "In my view," it would remind us that there are competing views. (Of course, some physicians already do this some of the time.) "Wait!" I can hear someone saying. "We want our doctors to be exact and certain of what they tell us." Yes, we do, but they aren't or shouldn't be nearly as certain as we want to believe, and it does us no good to imagine that they are when they are not. When we communicate with each other using impersonal, absolute language we are led into a naive realism where we come to think there is a single reality that we all share. This naive realism in turn leads us away from realizing that we have choices and enjoy possibility.

In fact, in several experiments my students and I found that when we substitute conditional terms such as *could be*, *perhaps*, or *in one view* for *is* people actually question the information and are able to think about it in new ways. In one of these studies we altered part of a textbook on urban development to read conditionally, in another we altered a programmed text on learning CPR to read conditionally, and in a third we showed them objects labeled either conditionally or absolutely—"This could be a dog's chew toy" or "This is a dog's chew toy"—and then tested participants on the creative use of the item.[1] Those participants for whom the information was presented as conditional were able to think about and use the information creatively in the future. If I tell you that a high cholesterol level is dangerous, stress is likely to follow. If we learned that a high level of cholesterol could be dangerous, we're probably going to be less stressed but more attentive to our health than if we were told nothing. Using conditional language leads both the speaker and the listener to be more mindful. Of course, we as listeners can and perhaps should hear conditionally regardless of how absolute the speaker is being. Moreover, by recognizing that language is not the same thing as experience and that it speaks to our similarities rather than our differences, we are more inclined to recognize that our health experience, although described similarly to others, may be quite unique. Only we know what our experience is and we cannot afford to give up our control of it. No matter how careful a doctor is, his role as expert, combined with a patient's expectation for certainty, make the language of medicine very powerful.

Recent research by psychologists Jean-François Bonnefon and Gaelle Villejoubert speaks to how we misinterpret doctors, even when they use words such as *possibly* to describe a patient's illness.[2] If your supervisor at work tells you, "You may possibly get to take a trip to Europe next summer," you're likely to imagine that even though the chances are slim, there is the possibility that you may get to actually go. But if she tells you, "Your raise will possibly be refused," you're more likely to think in certainties—it's not going to come through and she's just using *possibly* to soften the blow of the bad news. Bonnefon and Villejoubert found that in the case of minor side effects or ailments ("You may possibly suffer from muscle aches"), *possibly* is usually interpreted in the first sense: the doctor is not sure that it will happen and the chances are just as good that you might not suffer muscle aches. When side effects or medical conditions are mentioned less absolutely ("You may go deaf"), however, the interpretation is more likely to be that the doctor is sure that it will happen, but he is trying to be tactful. Patients who interpret it in this way imagine that they are very likely to contract the ailment, whatever the degree of probability the doctor actually has in mind, which can lead to irrational decisions about what action to take. The point is that sometimes conditional language is understood as absolute and sometimes not. It's important that we understand that conditional language doesn't guarantee a conditional understanding of our diseases.

Some people believe we have power over our diseases but they nonetheless unwittingly accept metaphors that may work against them. Instead of giving in to disease, we encourage ourselves to try to "fight" it. That's an interesting word choice, one that feels quite dramatic but might incur hidden effects. If a very young child were annoying us, we would not "fight" the child; we only fight worthy opponents. Thus the idea of battling and fighting illness only bolsters the power we feel it has over our health. We may well be better off with another metaphor, such as mastering our condition, which implies learning everything we can about it in order to control it over the long haul. The words we use matter.

Priming and Placebos

Add the following numbers up: one thousand plus forty, plus one thousand, plus thirty, plus one thousand, plus twenty, plus one thousand, plus ten. Many people come up with five thousand as the answer to this problem, given to us by Shlomo Benartzi of UCLA Anderson School of Management. The repetition of the word *thousand* primes us to think in thousands. The correct answer, however, is not 5,000, but 4,100. We're often unaware of our errors.

Most of us think that we are in charge of our thoughts and can choose to direct them one way or another. If we learn the information mindfully, this will be the case. Much of what we have learned, however, was learned mindlessly as we uncritically accepted information without thinking about it, often because the information was given to us by an authority or was initially irrelevant. Even if it is to our advantage to rethink the information at some point, it simply doesn't occur to us to do so. This makes us very vulnerable to the effects of priming, which we saw in the previous chapter. The way priming works is to trigger ideas we have mindlessly committed ourselves to without our awareness. For example, if we've learned that women are not very good at math, and the concept "woman" is primed, math ability will suffer. Psychologists Margaret Shih, Todd Pittinsky, and Nalini Ambady found just this when they had female Asian students take math tests where for one group their identity of "Asian" was primed and for another group their identity as "woman" was primed.[3] The stereotype of Asians is that they are good in math. The stereotype of women is that they are not good in math. They primed gender by asking questions such as whether they lived in a coed dorm. They primed ethnic identity by asking if there were any languages other than English spoken in their extended family. Their scores plunged when their identities as women were primed, but when their identities as Asians were primed, their scores soared.

We find primes everywhere in our lives and culture—a casual comment, the crossword puzzle we are filling in, a billboard, or a television program. No matter how inconsequential it may seem, a single word can lead us to behave in ways we would have rejected if only we were more aware of what was happening.

We have learned so much about physical and psychological health and health-related matters mindlessly that vast amounts of information can be primed with very little provocation. Psychologist Becca Levy found that when seniors were primed for positive stereotypes of aging, their memory and self-reliance in remembering improved, and when they were primed with negative cues, their memory and self-reliance in remembering grew worse.[4] What most influenced their response was the degree of importance that they put on the stereotypes for their self-image. Those who were more sensitive to the negative stereotypes activated fears within themselves and impaired their memory and self-reliance in remembering. Levy had participants sit at a computer that was programmed to present descriptions of behavior that were related to positive images ("see all sides of issues") or negative ones ("can't recall birthdays") faster than they could make out the words. Afterward, they were given a memory test and a test of their attitudes toward aging. The latter test presented participants with situations that could be interpreted in at least two ways—for example, one about a seventy-three-year-old woman who moved in with her daughter. Those who interpreted the situation negatively saw the older woman as dependent, and those who interpreted the situation positively saw her as interdependent. Participants who were initially primed with positive words showed memory improvements over control groups; similarly, when primed with negative words, they performed worse.

Another study conducted by Becca Levy with Jeffrey Hausdorff, Rebecca Hencke, and Jeanne Wei showed that priming individuals for health can activate healthy behavior, just as wisdom-related words primed a healthier memory.[5] Participants completed a "language proficiency task" that activated thoughts about a healthy lifestyle or an unhealthy lifestyle. Those who were primed for a healthy lifestyle were more likely to use the stairs instead of the elevator later. Simply priming "health" can facilitate healthy behavior. Studies such as these seem to suggest that mindlessness can be a good thing in that it enables positive primes to affect us so easily. The problem is that the unconscious influence of primes also takes a toll on us. When we are mindless, we can't control their effects.

This can be seen in the recent explosion of healthy fast-food products. McDonald's now offers several salad options as well as yogurt and granola for dessert. Fast-food restaurants as a category, however, prime us for the burgers and fries. Despite the healthy food on the menu, the name McDonald's, the smell of the burgers, and all the other things that we associate with fast food can prime us to eat burgers and fries instead of the healthier fare. In a study assessing people's attitudes toward food, researchers found that the environment does prime participants to make certain mindless associations with food; when their attention was focused on how good the food tastes, they preferred food such as burgers and fries.[6] Similarly, when participants were focused on health, participants displayed a preference for healthier foods and a greater preference for low-fat versus high-fat foods. The study also found that increasing levels of craving made them hungrier and less interested in health-related benefits and encouraged selecting and eating foods solely based on taste. McDonald's has been in the business of burgers and fries forever, so it is reasonable that people will associate it with unhealthy fast food. Adding salads and healthier fare may diminish critics of supersized portions, but it not likely to greatly improve our eating habits. As these researchers point out, our food choices often depend on whether we are walking through a street lined with nice restaurants and filled with the smell of tasty food or whether we are walking past a fitness gym or an advertisement for beachwear right before we sit down to eat.

In a wonderfully interesting study, researchers Baba Shiv, Ziv Carmon, and Dan Ariely gave participants at a fitness center what they were led to believe was an energy-enhancing drink before beginning their regular workouts.[7] One group was told that the cost of the drink was $2.89. Another group was told that the drink regularly sold for $2.89, but because they bought it in bulk, the discounted price was just 89 cents. Those in the "reduced price" group rated their workout intensity as lower and reported that they were more fatigued afterward than the "regular price" group. More expensive may often mean better, but in cases like these the expensive prime is unnecessarily costly.

In another clever study Dan Ariely, Baba Shiv, and Rebecca L. Waber conducted on placebos, a drug was described as a new "opioid analgesic," approved by the Food and Drug Administration, that was supposed to work like codeine but faster.[8] Half of their participants were told the drug cost $2.50 a pill and half were told it had been discounted to 10 cents. The researchers found that when the pill was presented as more expensive, it was more effective in reducing pain, despite the fact that everyone received the same placebo.

Price aside, placebos may be the best example of primes. We presume a pill is going to make us better, and thus it primes health, even though the pill contains an inert substance. Asking how placebos work means that we are essentially asking how we get from our thoughts to our bodies. If we conceive of the mind as a separate entity from the body, then to understand such phenomena as placebos, we need to figure out how they communicate with each other. Mind and body have not always been seen as separate, however. There have been periods of history and cultures in which this dualism is not an assumption. Today, in fact, among the !Kung, the people of the Kalahari Desert of southern Africa, mind and body are still considered one: healing practices for physical and psychological disturbances are the same. Their all-night healing dances are performed to treat problems ranging from marital problems to coughs to insufficient breast milk. The healing energy of the community is focused on the whole person, not simply the mind or the body. It's unfortunate that only among an isolated tribe like this do we still see this nondualism.

In psychology, a dualistic view of mind and body has been very persistent. Until the end of the last century, psychology was a branch of philosophy and took its notions of mind from those held by philosophers. The separation of mind and body is often traced to Descartes, who thought the mind was nonmaterial and the body was material. Only the body was subject to the laws of physics. Though many have tried to dispel that kind of thinking, most of us still look at ourselves in this dualist way.

All this is not a matter of semantics or academic theorizing; the separation of mind and body has serious consequences. The distinctions we make between physical and mental illness are questionable. We shouldn't separate them or try to reduce one to the other, nor should they be thought to be distinct but "related" entities.

The psychologist Herbert Lefcourt tells the story of an institutionalized woman who had been in a mute state for nearly ten years when she and others in her unit were moved to a different floor of the building while their own was being renovated.[9] The third-floor unit where she had been living was known among the patients as the "chronic/hopeless" floor. Her new unit, on the first floor, usually held patients who were close to being released and enjoyed special privileges, including the freedom to wander the hospital grounds and the neighboring streets.

Prior to moving the patients, staff gave medical examinations to the patients, and the woman in question was judged to be in excellent medical health, despite being mute and withdrawn. Much to the surprise of her doctors, shortly after moving to the first floor and enjoying some of the first-floor privileges, the patient began to be responsive to the staff and other patients, and soon she began to speak, in time becoming quite gregarious. Unfortunately, the redecoration of the third floor was soon complete. Within a week after she had been returned to the "hopeless" unit, the woman collapsed and died. Her autopsy revealed no known medical cause, although some suggested that she had died of despair.

When we see mind and body as parts of a single entity, the research on placebos takes on new meaning and suggests we can not only control much of our disease experience, but we may also be able to extend our ability to gain, recover, or enhance our health.

Placebos often come in the form of a single word that captures a richer mindset. In one study I conducted with my students, we explored the mindset most of us have regarding the excellent vision air force pilots have.[10] All participants were given a vision test. One group of participants was then encouraged to role-play "air force pilots." They dressed the part and, in uniform, sat in a flight simulator. They were asked to read the letters on the wing of a nearby plane, which were actually part of an eye chart. Those participants who adopted the "pilot" mindset, primed to have excellent vision, showed improved vision over those who were simulating being in the simulator and simply asked to read an eye chart from the same distance.

Three members of my lab, Maja Djikic, Michael Pirson, and Arin Madenci, recently continued this work on vision with Rebecca Donohue at Simmons College Department of Nursing.[11] Eye charts are designed such that the larger letters are on the top, with the letters growing progressively smaller down the chart. Since eye tests are administered top to bottom, this inadvertently creates the expectation that at some point we will not be able to clearly read the letters. What would happen if the chart were reversed, with the smallest letters on top? Now the expectation would be different. In this case we would expect that soon we'd be able to see. Participants tested indeed showed enhanced vision using the redesigned chart, and they were able to read lines they couldn't see before on a standard eye chart. In all but one case, subjects could read the same number of small letters on a line on the reversed chart that was only visible on a line ten font sizes larger on the regular eye charts. Also interesting was that the subjects thought they did better on the normal chart. We're blind to what we don't expect.

Starting with the observation that people typically believe they can easily read the first few lines of an eye chart, we tried shifting the chart instead of reversing it. We created a chart that began with letters the size of those found a third of the way down a normal chart. We then measured how far down the chart subjects could read and found that they performed better than they did with a normal chart. Again, they were able to see letters that they couldn't see before.

When someone reports that he has less than perfect vision, say 20/40 vision, what does that mean? Is it really reasonable to expect that under all circumstances he will be able to see equally well or poorly, regardless of how tired, hungry, or angry he may be? Regardless of the context in which the object viewed appears? Is seeing a moving target the same as seeing a still object? Is seeing something in one color the same as seeing it in others? Is seeing something familiar the same as seeing something novel? In each case, I think not.

There may be many ways to improve our vision. Psychologists Daphne Bavelier and C. Shawn Green, in fact, found that the act of playing video games can improve visual skills.[12] Interestingly, they attribute the improvement to the uncertainty regarding what will happen—and when it will happen; when we don't know what to expect, we stay mindful.

If our expectations affect our vision in this unusual way, it also may be the case for our hearing. Tom Mikuckis, another member of my lab, set out to test this using the vision study as a guide. We used an "equal loudness contours and audiometry" hearing test, provided online by the University of New South Wales. Each participant was played two series of tones twice separated in time by one week. For one, tones were played from loudest to softest, as the volume was decreased in three jumps of six decibels. For the other, the tones were played from softest to loudest. Participants indicated each time they heard a tone. To make this similar to the vision study, where people from the start knew that the order of the chart was reversed, participants in the second week were told what to expect before they began. The order of the series was controlled to eliminate practice effects. We used trials where there were no sounds to make sure all responses were honest. As with the vision study, we found that in the soft to loud series people were able to hear one step down in volume when they had the expectation that soon they would be able to hear but not in the control series (without the expectation). Fourteen of the twenty-one participants showed this improvement when the series was soft to loud. Just as language acts as a prime, so too do our expectations. They can have a measurable influence on bodies, including our ability to see and hear.

The placebo effect extends much further than many of us realize. It comes in many forms: subjects exposed to fake poison ivy have developed real rashes, and people imbibing placebo caffeine have been shown to experience increased motor performance and heart rate (and other effects congruent with the subjects' beliefs about the effects of caffeine and not with its pharmacological effects). Herbert Benson and D. P. McCallie Jr. studied the effectiveness of several placebo-like treatments for angina pectoris (a type of severe chest pain) and found that when patients actually believed in the therapies, they were 70 percent to 90 percent effective, while for those people who showed some form of skepticism they were only 30 percent to 40 percent effective.[13] Psychologists Alan Roberts, Donald Kewman, Lisa Mercier, and

Mel Hovell looked at the effects of "undergoing" a glomectomy (a placebo surgery) for ulcer patients and found that the more the subject believed in the effectiveness of the treatment, the more effective it actually was.[14]

Irving Kirsch and Guy Sapirstein conducted an analysis of antidepressant medication and found that out of 2,318 studies analyzed, 25 percent of the patient responses were due to the actual drug effect, another 25 percent were due to the natural progression of depression, and 50 percent were due to the placebo effect.[15] Other studies suggest that up to 65 percent of drugs and other therapies prescribed by physicians may depend on placebo action for their effectiveness.[16]

While the placebo effect has proven to be incredibly powerful in aiding health, the effect implies a double-edged sword in the same way as primes. The placebo response can also work in reverse when negative expectations are confirmed by negative outcomes in the patient. This effect is the "nocebo" phenomenon. For example, in the context of a cancer diagnosis, a very common mindset for Americans is the conviction that cancer means death. A person diagnosed with cancer has an extremely hard time viewing himself as healthy, even if the cancer has not yet had any effect on bodily functions. Yet at the same time there are people walking around with undiagnosed cancer who consider themselves to be healthy. "Malignantly diagnosed" patients may go into a decline that has little to do with the actual course of the illness, illustrating that the mere expectation of death can accelerate its occurrence.

The most dramatic example of language acting as placebo can be found in the counterclockwise study. The study used language to prime the participants, asking the elderly men at the retreat to speak about the past in the present tense. With language placing the experimental groups' minds in a healthier place, their bodies followed suit.

Mindful Exercise

More recently, my student Ali Crum and I took this idea of "putting the mind in a healthy place" to have a positive effect on the body in a very different direction.[17] We were curious as to whether some or all of the health benefits attributed to exercise were actually a function of our mindsets regarding the health benefits of exercise. Before looking at the dramatic results we found, let's look at some of the recent findings regarding the benefits of exercise to help understand the potential importance of our findings.

Probably for several reasons, today, twenty-eight countries have healthy life expectancies that exceed those of the United States. (The highest is in Japan, which exceeds the United States by about five years.) How could we become a healthier culture? Many believe that if we were not so sedentary, we would be healthier. Systematic research on exercise and physical health began in the 1950s, focusing on occupational exertion. Dr. Jeremy Morris, first professor of social medicine at the London Hospital Medical College, and colleagues conducted the first formal, empirical study comparing the cardiovascular heath of double-decker bus drivers to conductors. The study found significant results indicating lower rates of heart disease for the conductors, who ran up and down the stairs, versus the drivers who sat all day. The study ignited a new flurry in medical research focusing on the health effects of exercise.[18]

Physical activity has been shown to reduce the risk of dying prematurely. It has been estimated that about 250,000 deaths per year in the United States are attributable to lack of regular physical activity. Indeed, several longitudinal, correlational studies have indicated that the mortality rate is higher in people who report less physical activity or who have significantly lower baseline levels of cardiovascular fitness.[19] These studies are only suggestive since they were not controlled experiments. That being said, one study indicated that among middle-aged Harvard male alumni who were sedentary in 1962, those who took up moderately intense sports as physical activity during the study's eleven-year follow-up had a 23 percent lower death rate.[20] More recently, a study investigated seven thousand men and women ages twenty-nine to seventy-nine and found that increasing the amount of physical activity from low to moderate was associated with a reduced risk of death.[21] Lower risks of diabetes, cancer, coronary heart disease, high blood pressure, osteoarthritis, and obesity-related diseases have all been shown to have been associated with exercise. Similar findings now exist for psychological issues such as stress and depression. It certainly looks like exercise matters.

In 1995, after an extensive review of the literature, the Centers for Disease Control (CDC) issued new guidelines for all Americans: every adult should get thirty minutes or more of moderate-intensity physical activity on most, preferably all, days of the week.[22]

Studies suggest that physical activity doesn't need to be all in one session but can be accumulated throughout the day to be beneficial. While the exact amounts are debatable, the minimal or reasonable amount of exercise is approximately 150 kilocalories/day, which can be achieved by any of several activities, such as thirty minutes of walking or raking leaves, or fifteen minutes of running. Secretary of Health and Human Services Donna E. Shalala, in her foreword to the report, summed up the new guidelines by saying that we don't have to train like professional athletes to enjoy the benefits of exercise. Everyday activities such as walking, bicycling, or even tending a garden for at least thirty minutes per day most days of the week are good for our health.

Physical activity alters many different pathways—metabolic, hormonal, neurological, and mechanical—affecting virtually every tissue in the body. The report summarized the results from five surveys that provided data on national levels of physical activity. The conclusions were as follows:

- Approximately 15 percent of U.S. adults engage regularly (three times a week for at least twenty minutes) in vigorous physical activity during leisure time.

- Approximately 22 percent of adults engage regularly (five times a week for thirty minutes) in sustained physical activity of any intensity during leisure time.

- About 25 percent of adults report no physical activity in their leisure time.

- Physical inactivity is more prevalent among women than men, among blacks and Hispanics than whites, among older than younger adults, and among the less affluent than the most affluent.

- The most popular leisure-time physical activities among adults are walking and gardening or yard work.

One reason that America appears to be so sedentary is that the tools we are using to measure exercise fail to take into account all types of physical activity. To an increasingly white-collar workforce, exercise consists of activity done outside of work. Since the measures were created by white-collar workers, they didn't think of work as exercise. For example, the surveys used in the CDC report on prevalence of physical activity in 1996 included leisure-time physical activity and intentional exercise but failed to take into account household, family care, or transportation-type activities, which may explain why fewer women met the criteria than men. They also omitted occupational exercise, which may explain why Hispanics, blacks, and the less affluent fail to get sufficient "exercise" (since most of them have physically demanding jobs and have little time or energy to exercise after work). The data suggest that they need exercise. On the other hand, if we can prime the idea of exercise, can these people benefit without actually changing their daily habits? Can the idea of exercise act as a placebo?

Although many people today have sedentary jobs, there are some jobs in which people are getting plenty of physical activity throughout the course of their work. Hotel room attendants, for example, clean on average fifteen rooms a day, each taking between twenty and thirty minutes to complete and requiring such exertion as pushing, reaching, bending, and lifting. Room attendants are therefore meeting or exceeding the surgeon general's requirements for a healthy lifestyle. Yet despite their levels of activity, descriptive statistics reveal that the health of these women is exceedingly poor. Room attendants appear at risk with respect to blood pressure, body mass index, body fat percentage, total body water percentage, and waist-to-hip ratio, all important indicators of health.

Room attendants also tend to have the mindless view that exercise and work are distinct and separate activities, which provides an opportunity to see whether they can get the health benefits of exercise if we prime exercise. When Ali Crum and I decided to study this group in 2007, we determined that these women did not initially view their work as exercise. At the outset of the experiment, two-thirds of them reported not exercising regularly, and around one-third reported not getting any exercise at all. If we change the attitudes of room attendants who are getting the required amount of physical activity but do not perceive it as exercise, will they reap the benefits?

We first asked how healthy female room attendants are, in general. What is the relationship between their physical activity and their actual health? Further we asked, "Are room attendants aware that their work is a good source of daily exercise?" Seven hotels helped us study these questions, and each was randomly assigned to one of the following two conditions.

In the informed group, to make room attendants aware that they are getting a sufficient amount of exercise at work to reap its benefits, participants in this condition received a notice discussing the benefits of exercise and were informed that their daily housekeeping work satisfies the CDC's recommendations for an active lifestyle. This notice, written in both English and Spanish, was read and explained to the participants by an experimenter unaware of the hypotheses and then posted on the information bulletin board in their lounge.

Participants were told that we were interested in getting information on their health so that we could study ways to improve it. In return for helping, we would give them information about our research on health and happiness. They had no knowledge that the information was related to the physiological measures taken.

The control group was treated in the same way as the informed group except they did not receive information about work as exercise (although we later told them this information, after the second set of measures was taken).

Participants for the study were recruited through the hotels. We began the study by taking several health measures including weight and blood pressure. To prevent participants in different experimental groups from sharing information, all room attendants within a hotel were put in the same condition. In total, there were eighty-four participants.

In a one-hour session, all participants were told that we were interested in studying ways to improve the health and happiness of women in a hotel workplace. They were each given a questionnaire to complete. While the women began filling out the questionnaire, they were individually taken to another room to complete their physiological measures. Following this, the experimental group was given a short presentation on how their work is good exercise, similar to workouts that people do at the gym. Four weeks later, we returned to take follow-up measures. We asked all the questions we could think of to see if participants changed their actual behavior over the course of the study. Participants also were asked to report how hard they perceived themselves to be working compared to other housekeepers.

What did we find? The experimental group increased their perceived exercise over the course of the study, whereas the control group did not. The percentage of informed participants who reported that they were receiving regular exercise more than doubled. All but one person in the experimental group reported getting at least some exercise. Neither group, however, increased their actual exercise.

Now that we knew the instructions were understood, how did they do?

This shift in mindset from the lack of awareness of exercise to exercise was accompanied by a remarkable improvement in physiological health. After only four weeks of knowing that their work is good exercise, the participants in the informed group lost an average of two pounds. In addition to the weight loss, the room attendants also showed a significant reduction in body fat percentage. Further, the fact that the participants in the informed condition showed an increase in body water percentage indicates, first, that they did not simply lose water weight and, second, that they may have gained some muscle mass (muscle mass has a higher water content than fatty tissue), making the 2.7 percent loss even more significant (since muscle weighs more than fat). Finally, the fact that these were significant differences between the informed group and the control group, who were actually gaining weight and body fat, makes these findings even more powerful. With respect to blood pressure, the informed group showed a drop of 10 points systolic and 5 points diastolic in their blood pressure—a significant change.

While there may be numerous reasons why the women in the study may have been unhealthy, including genetics and diet, our study focused on exercise. These women did not initially view their work as exercise. At the onset of the experiment, two-thirds of the participants reported not exercising regularly, and around one-third reported not getting any exercise at all.

It is important to note that while the informed room attendants did report getting more exercise, they did not report getting any additional exercise outside of work. There was actually a decrease in reported physical activity outside of work, including such activities as running, swimming, or doing sit-ups. The room attendants did not walk more often on the way to work and did not pick up any other jobs that required cleaning or manual labor. In addition, information provided by their supervisors indicated that their daily work level remained consistent throughout the course of the experiment. The changes in reported physical activity are attributable not to actual increases in physical activity but to a shift in mindset initiated by the information given to them in the intervention.

According to conventional science, it is assumed that in order for weight loss and body fat reduction to take place, certain biological and physiological events must also take place. In the case of blood pressure, it is assumed that during exercise blood pressure is lowered because the peripheral blood vessels are dilated, and over time, the attenuating effect of exercise on the sympathetic nervous system activity helps to control blood pressure. In the case of weight, it is assumed that exercise helps to reduce body fat by increasing nonresting energy expenditure. To the extent that energy expenditure exceeds caloric intake the result is weight loss; theoretically, about one pound of fat energy is lost for each additional 3,500 kilocalories burned. If this is indeed the case, how did the change in mindset (increase in perceived exercise) initiate these physiological changes?

Skeptics will argue that despite our results, the connection between perceived exercise and health was moderated by a change in behavior. For example, a change in mindset may have given the informed participants an incentive to change their habits with respect to diet and substance abuse. Previous research, however, has found it very difficult to change behavior of this sort. If it did, that too would make these results interesting. Instead, given the plethora of research on the difficulty of changing such behavior and given the fact that participants in this study reported no such change, it seems that the explanation is that health follows a change in mindset just as in the case with placebos.

The search for explanations for findings such as these results from mind/body dualism that simply denies the direct influence of the mind on the body. This dualism has left us with few conceptual tools to aid us in understanding and explaining undeniable occurrences such as the placebo effect. Despite the fact that traditional medical models typically do not allow for the unity of mind and body, few deny the fact that stressors, sexual stimuli, fear, and disgust reactions manifest in bodily reactions. Our mindsets regarding illness and well-being can occasion powerful effects on our physiology.

As to what was happening simultaneously on the physiological level in our hotel room attendant study, we do not know. While having an explanation on that level is appealing, it does not speak to what we can do ourselves to improve our health. An interesting study by Deena Skolnick Weisberg, Frank C. Keil, Joshua Goodstein, Elizabeth Rawson, and Jeremy R. Gray is important here.[23] The title of their paper tells it all: "The Seductive Allure of Neuroscience Explanations." The researchers presented a set of research findings to students in a cognitive neuroscience class and to people with no neuroscience background, asking them to judge how good the explanation for the finding was. When the explanation contained irrelevant references to neuroscience—phrases such as "because of frontal lobe brain circuitry"—the participants found the results more believable than when they did not.

Although we haven't done the research, one might ask, what would happen with people who perceive themselves as exercisers but are actually not getting exercise? I feel healthier when I set out to get exercise even if in fact I spend little time actually moving. In truth, I see time away from the refrigerator as exercise, but that is a separate matter. Do our thoughts about food actually determine the effect it will have on our bodies? For example, do those who do not lose weight from sugar substitutes essentially believe they are consuming sugar? If we imagined eating candy, would our blood sugar increase? Do our thoughts about clean air actually affect our ability to breathe? Do our thoughts about contagion actually affect our getting sick?

Many people these days elect to have plastic surgery. If we put the ideas of the experiments just described together, we end up with an interesting idea: if I think I look younger, I should be younger on whatever measures of age we take. Further, I may now exercise more, which may have added benefits. I probably will also think I am getting more exercise because younger people simply do. Vanity in this case, then, may pay off.

Psychologists Gerald Davison and Stuart Valins conducted a study back in the 1970s where people were given shocks and the researchers kept track of how much pain they were willing to take.[24] They were then given a pill (a placebo) and told it would make them better able to withstand the shock. The machine administering the shocks was rigged so it appeared that everyone was able to withstand more shock than they were actually being subjected to. Then half of the subjects were told that it was actually a placebo that they had taken. The other half were told that the effects of the pill had worn off. All were retested to see how much shock they could take. The group told they had taken a placebo now attributed their greater performance to themselves rather than the pill and as a result, they were able to withstand more shock. If we gave a person a placebo for their health symptoms and the symptoms disappeared and then we told her it was a placebo, she would know that she was actually responsible for the improvement. Would it generalize? I think so. What would we do differently? I think we would tune in to and try to use the subtle messages our bodies give us.

It is a widely known fact that placebos are effective in treating a vast number of disorders. When a study finds that medication resulted in, say, a 90 percent improvement and the placebo gave only a 30 percent improvement, the drug is seen as effective. What is missing from these studies is a comparison of the side effects. Placebos have no negative side effects, while the side effects for most drugs are significant. Surely it is more than worthwhile to figure out how to harness the potent effects of more benign substances. In fact, do we really need the placebo pills at all?

Placebos are wonderful things, it seems. We accept a pill along with the lie that it is effective, and so we adopt a beneficial mindset and heal ourselves (it can't be the pill, after all, because it is a placebo). And then attribute the success to the pill. Wouldn't it be more advantageous to recognize that when placebos work we are the ones controlling our health, to learn how to exercise it directly, and to see ourselves as efficacious when we do?

Social psychologists are fond of saying that behavior is largely a function of the contexts in which we find ourselves. We behave differently, for example, in libraries than we do at football games. Contexts serve as primes. What few have addressed, however, is who controls the context. Since situations can be viewed in many different ways, and situations control our behavior, we can choose the view that supports how we want to be. There are what we can call healthy contexts and those that are less so.

Laura Hsu, Jaewoo Chung, and I collected archival data to

provide further evidence of the effects of our minds over our bodies.[25] This work also suggests a way to begin taking more direct control of our health. Negative stereotypes about aging, as we have seen, may directly and indirectly prime diminished capacity for older adults. Similarly, the absence of these cues may prime improved health. The general hypothesis examined here was that if we are in contexts that prime older age, we will age more quickly. We examined the effect that our clothes may have on us given the age-appropriate stance we take on clothing. Imagine a sixty-year-old woman trying on a miniskirt. In most cases, she'd be well advised not to make the purchase, but we would think nothing of a sixteen-year-old wearing the same skirt.

Since uniforms are less age-related than everyday clothing, we reasoned that people who wear uniforms are not exposed to as many age-related cues as those who wear their own clothes to work. As a result, we expect the absence of these cues would be related to better health. We examined morbidity data from 206 professions from the National Health Interview Survey conducted between 1986 and 1994. We found that those who wear uniforms do have better health, as indicated by fewer lost days from work due to illness or injury, doctor visits, hospitalizations, self-reported health status, and chronic conditions, when compared to those who earn the same amount of money and do not wear uniforms.

We next considered whether clothing serves as an even greater age-related cue for the middle and upper-middle classes. We reasoned that if wealthier people wear clothes that are more varied and change their wardrobe more frequently because they can afford it, they should experience more age-related cues. Thus the uniform effect should become more prominent at higher income levels. Indeed, we found that wealthier individuals who *do not* wear work uniforms have poorer health than their uniformed counterparts, and the effect was greater as we looked higher up the income spectrum.

A count of the number of different brands and styles of jeans and shirts at Nordstrom, a high-end department store, and Sears, a less expensive department store, revealed a significant difference. While Nordstrom had thirty-eight different brands of jeans and ten different leg styles (i.e., boot cut, flare), Sears featured seventeen jean brands and five leg styles. Nordstrom had 930 styles of shirts compared to 560 styles at Sears. The greater selection of clothing at Nordstrom suggests there are more buying options for people with more earning potential. Since clothing is a status symbol, having more money means having the purchasing power to keep up with constantly changing trends in fashion. For those in the higher income levels, a uniform may act as a "buffer" for being all too aware of one's age.

We also examined premature balding to test this idea. Baldness is a cue for old age. Therefore, men who go bald early in life may perceive themselves as older and are consequently predicted to age more quickly. We found that men who bald prematurely have a greater risk of being diagnosed with prostate cancer and of getting coronary heart disease than men who are not bald. When I describe this finding to people they assume that the result is due to some hormonal difference between the men who bald prematurely and those who don't. Yet when we asked several medical specialists about their understanding of a relationship between premature balding and prostate cancer, none of them could explain it.

Next we looked at women who bear children later in life, believing that they are surrounded by younger cues and thus are expected to live longer. We found older mothers have a longer life expectancy than women who bear children early in life. Given the wear and tear of raising children on a parent of any age, you might expect the opposite here.

Finally, we compared marriages in which spouse's ages differed by more than four years to those with a lesser age difference. In the former, the younger spouses are surrounded by "older" cues provided by the older spouse, and thus we predicted them to have shorter life spans. Conversely, older spouses are primed by "younger" cues by the younger spouse and thus we predicted they would have longer life spans. As predicted, we found that spouses who are significantly younger than their partner have shorter life expectancies than spouses who are much older than their partner.

It seems that certain contexts typically cue age. If we are in these contexts, we could choose to attend to those cues that best serve us, rather than be mindlessly led to be less than we can be.

The effect of being in one context or another may also be relevant to physiological states. Consider the degree to which fatigue may be a psychological construct. If contextual cues signal that we "should" be tired, we may experience more fatigue than we would if they did not signal exhaustion. Many years ago, my students and I tested this hypothesis informally. People in class asked their friends to do either 100 or 200 jumping jacks and asked them to tell us when they got tired. Both groups reported that they experienced fatigue two-thirds of the way through the activity. That means that the first group got tired after about 65–70 jumping jacks but the second group after about 130–140. In another experiment, we had people type one or two pages in a word-processing program that gave them no feedback regarding errors, so they would type the assignment continuously. For the one-page group, the most errors occurred around two-thirds of the way through. Although the second group typed twice as much, their errors didn't appear until two-thirds of the way through the two pages.

What's going on here? I think we impose a structure on the tasks we do so that we have a sense of a beginning, a middle, and an end. Feeling ourselves grow tired as we near the finish of a task may make it easier for us to leave it so that we can begin the next task. Perhaps people who can't seem to "get on with things" have a poorly developed or nonexistent structure of the task they are doing.

Everyday examples of the psychological aspect of fatigue abound. Consider the end of the workday, when we may feel we are running out of energy, only to go home and have a night on the town. Indeed, the 3:00 P.M. coffee break may be a result of this "two-thirds effect." Be that as it may, the larger point is that much of what we take to be physical limits may be a result of learning. We've learned concepts such as beginning, middle, and end, and our bodies behave accordingly.

CHAPTER 7

What's in a Word?

Where is the wisdom we lost in knowledge?

—T. S. Eliot, *The Rock*

In 1979, at the age of fifty-six, my mother died of breast cancer. At least, that's what the medical world reported. I'm still not sure. Before she died, her cancer had gone into "complete remission." Had another cancer developed in her body quickly, or was it the same cancer back to haunt her? To this day, I don't know what *remission* really means. Psychologically, however, *remission* suggests something very different from *cure*. Language has the interesting property of being able to increase and decrease our perceptions of control. Different word choices can direct our thoughts about a single situation in many different ways. If somebody has cancer and the cancer goes away, we say it is in remission. The implication is that the same cancer may recur. If that same cancer does not return, was it in "remission," or has it actually been "cured"?

Now, contrast the language of cancer with that of a cold. We tend to speak of each cold we catch as a new cold. Each time we beat a cold, we become more persuaded that we can beat the next one. While there are surely similarities among the various colds we have had over the course of our lifetimes, there are also many differences from one cold to the next. "This time it started with a sore throat; last time it started with a stuffy nose." Most of us are quite good at analyzing the progress of colds, but who decided we should pay attention to the differences—as most of us do— and not the similarities? Most of us are oblivious to the idea that there is any choice involved. We were simply led early on in life to believe that each new cold is different from the last but we can master them all. The psychological evidence for this is that our last cold left us at some point. We were successful at beating it.

With respect to cancer, however, being in "remission" means that we are waiting for "it" to return. If "it" does return, the re- currence is seen as part of the same cancer. Psychologically, this may lead us to feel defeated. For each new cold we beat, we im- plicitly think, "I beat it before, so I can beat it again." If the can- cer comes back, however, we think, " 'It' is winning. I am just not as strong as 'it' is." Surely the cancer will in some ways bear a similarity to the last cancer, but in other ways, it is just as surely different. Our language leads us to see the similarities in recur- ring episodes of cancer, while with the common cold we see the dissimilarities. Of course, the stakes are so much higher with cancer that there is even more reason to consider our language choices.

Ever since my mother's death, I've been somewhat ambiva- lent about the medical world. I have turned to medical doctors when seriously ill, yet I think many underestimate the power of psychology to influence health. As we have seen, the psychological literature is replete with examples of the physical consequences of giving up. Even if one were not as persuaded by the experimental data as I am, it is clear that giving up affects health choices and keeps people from wanting to survive. Why exercise or take medication if one is likely to die soon anyway? Did cancer kill my mother, or did the language that we use to describe cancer lead her to give up?

A friend of mine was diagnosed with breast cancer, which is now in "remission." She has every reason to believe that she is now fine, but even so, she is scared. When we talk about her cancer, all of the events surrounding my mother's death vividly return to me. Would things have turned out differently if my mother had thought that her second episode of cancer was not identical to the first? Would my friend be more at ease now if we used the word *cure* rather than *remission* to describe her state?

My colleagues Aline Flodr, Shelley Carson, and I recently looked into the effects of language on the well-being of cancer survivors.[1] We recruited sixty-four women from around New England who were participating in events such as the Race for a Cure and Making Strides walking events, women who had been treated for breast cancer but were now in a stable condition. We gave them several health questionnaires and a mindfulness scale to complete. One question asked them in which of two categories they would place themselves: in remission or cured. After we analyzed the results, we found that the "cured" group reported significantly higher general health, better physical functioning, fewer role limitations due to health, and less pain. There was also a tendency for them to experience more energy and less fatigue. Regarding their emotional health, they reported greater well-being and social functioning and were significantly less depressed.

When we looked at scores on the mindfulness scale, irrespective of whether they saw themselves as cured, we found that the more mindful a woman was, the better her physical functioning was, the more energy she had, the greater her overall well-being was, and the fewer limitations she had due to her emotional health. All in all, the results were impressive.

The same kinds of issues about language arise in the simple difference between characterizing an alcoholic as "recovering" instead of "recovered." If an alcoholic has not had a drink in ten years, it seems odd to characterize that person as still recovering. The word *recovering* suggests that we are victims and helpless against our conditions.

We are told that alcoholics should view themselves as recovering instead of recovered, to remind them that they should not drink. It may be easier, however, to refrain from drinking when one feels strong. *Recovering* suggests that you've never quite beaten the problem. *Recovered* suggests conviction and strength. It seems to me that the stronger one feels, the less likely one is to revert to harmful behaviors.

What if we called alcoholism an allergy instead of a disease? If one had a severe allergy to alcohol, he or she might think twice about drinking. People who are allergic to shellfish typically don't eat shrimp or mollusks. The word *allergy* suggests that the person who is allergic is in charge of treating it; the word *disease* offers much less control.

A new look at the language of medicine could have far-ranging implications. If I take Prozac or Paxil, for example, my depressive symptoms may go away, but I still describe myself as a depressed person. I am likely to attribute most of the relief I experience to the medication, but the misery always remains mine. If I take an aspirin to treat a headache, however, I believe my headache has "gone away," even if I am regularly prone to headaches and likely to suffer another.

If antidepressants are effective in removing depression just as aspirin works to remove headaches, it seems to me that people on antidepressants should not see themselves as being depressed any longer. If there are no symptoms of depression, then it follows that there should be no depression, despite the fact that antidepressants are still being taken.

The labels we choose to apply may have positive as well as negative effects. Consider vitamins. Even though they come in pill form and may be taken to alleviate problems such as arthritis and fatigue, they are nonetheless thought of as "vitamins." While we take "vitamins" to stay healthy, we take "pills" when we are sick. To my mind, "to be healthy" is not the same thing as "not to be sick." Each time someone says they're taking a vitamin, their perception of being healthy gets a boost. To take a "pill," in contrast, may reinforce my perception of being ill.

We ought to consider using language to repackage our experience of our health and illness. The word *painkiller* implicitly reinforces the idea that we have no choice in how we interpret certain sensations. Pain, it seems is something to kill. To kill it suggests that it is a very big problem indeed and we are helpless without pills; instead we could take pain pills to erase the pain, rather than kill it. Be that as it may, "pain" consists of many different sensations. Instead of one big problem to be killed with pills, we could interpret pain simply as sensations. There may be an advantage to not naming our sensations but merely to experience them. If we did, we would see that they don't stand still. They change. A headache may throb at one point while the sensations are barely noticeable the next. To notice the changes gives us a chance to control the sensations. Noticing the changes may also lead us to not need to exert any control. After all, the pain may subside on its own.

The way we use language encourages people with cancer, alcoholism, or depression to consider their disorders as an intractable part of who they are. Colds and headaches, by contrast, describe how we are at a particular time, not who we are. We might be able to improve "how we are" if we make decisions about what to call our ailments based on the differences from one episode to the next. If I enter the physician's office with stomach pains, for example, I leave feeling somewhat better knowing I have "gastroenteritis." Having a name for our disorders gives us some comfort. We have much more control, however, once we realize that a particular name and its implications are just one of several that could have been chosen. If it was not serious, it could have been indigestion, among other things; if serious, it could have been a result of an ulcer. Most of us remain oblivious to that choice.

The choices available to us become clear when we find ourselves in situations in which words are used differently than we are accustomed to, or when someone describes the same situation in which we find ourselves in a different way. Years ago, I tried a new dictation program for my computer. I had injured the middle finger of my right hand and, to get on with my writing, I decided to dictate it to the computer. When I spoke about my "gastroenteritis," the phrase "Castro decided to invite us" appeared on the screen. When I spoke about a "belief," it took me on a trip to "Belize." The voice recognition software was programmed to suggest words without awareness of their context. We, however, can be aware of context and ought to choose language very carefully, especially when our health is involved.

We have a choice whether to see ourselves as in remission or cured, to call alcoholism an allergy or a disease—to open up the labels that describe our conditions to see what actually lies beneath the name.

Mindless or Mindful Labels

To be fair, labels help us organize our thoughts. The problems begin, however, when they determine our thoughts. Although we can learn labels deliberately or blindly, all too often it is the latter, which often results in what I've termed "premature cognitive commitments." More simply, we mindlessly accept labels as fixed truths.

I've been studying the negative effects of premature cognitive commitments, or mindsets, for over thirty years. When colleague Benzion Chanowitz and I studied premature cognitive commitments we found that when we take in information without questioning it, we implicitly make a commitment to a single understanding of the information we have accepted.[2] We treat it as true and it never occurs to us to question it, even if it would be to our advantage to do so. We often take in information we deem irrelevant in just this way. After all, why bother thinking about it if it isn't important? The problem is that what may be irrelevant at one time may later become quite relevant. We take in information about diseases such as cancer or dementia when we are young and imagine that we will live a very long, healthy life. Later, when forced to confront them, the labels we applied can catch up with us and lead us to places we wouldn't want to go if we stayed in charge.

In this research, Chanowitz and I invented a disorder that we called "chromosythosis," which we explained could lead to diminished hearing. We told the participants we were going to test them for the disorder and gave them a booklet describing its symptoms. We did not, however, give everyone identical materials. Three of the four groups we worked with were given booklets that stated that 80 percent of the population had the disorder, which was meant to make the possibility of having the disorder more relevant. We also asked them to imagine how they might help themselves if they were diagnosed as having chromosythosis. The fourth group was given booklets that told them the disorder was rare, only 10 percent of the population had it, making the disease less relevant to them. We didn't ask them to consider how they might deal with a diagnosis, all of which we hypothesized would lead them to process the information mindlessly.

They did, indeed. We gave all of them a "hearing test" for chromosythosis, which confirmed they indeed had the disorder, and then a series of follow-up tests for specific disabilities described in the booklets. Those for whom the disorder was less relevant, the mindless readers, performed less than half as well as the other groups on the specific follow-up tests than those who thought the material and our instructions to think about how to deal with it were more relevant to them. The way they first processed the information determined how they later used it.

Cognitive commitments can come in the form of a word to describe a single symptom or disease and can be deadly. Even as science is learning that cancer can be a chronic condition or even fully treatable, most of us mindlessly process the label that cancer is a "killer." If later diagnosed with cancer, we may be more prone to give up, having accepted that our cancer is a killer, when the course of any particular cancer could be otherwise.

How many people trying and failing to have a baby are labeled "infertile"? The label makes the condition stable when for some it may not be. Once labeled infertile, the extreme disappointment may lead to depression and stress—neither of which is good for a relationship (and some doctors think that stress itself is a contributing factor to infertility). If the relationship suffers, sex may diminish, and with that the likelihood of conception decreases, making the diagnosis, in this example, a self-fulfilling prophecy.

Traditional medicine is characterized by a stepwise process involving a patient's symptoms, the doctor's diagnosis, and a subsequent treatment. Even before the diagnosis, the labeling begins. The patient is "one who receives medical attention, care, or treatment." The patient is also defined as "one who suffers." Soon the patient will acquire more labels; she will be identified as having "illness X," the symptoms of which will be described further as "acute" or "mild." The doctor may tell you that the treatment may be "risky." These labels can be detrimental to both the patient and the future of medicine.

Doctors have been trained in the art of clinical diagnosis using language as a tool to classify particular sets of symptoms. Through the act of classification, the agent assumes control over what he is labeling. For example, in the diagnostic process, doctors may feel reassured professionally for having matched a certain set of symptoms to a specific illness. In naming the disease, the diagnostician has placed the uncertain, unpredictable symptoms of the disease beneath a comforting, familiar name tag. He feels secure, as though he had regained control over the menacing microbes. Diagnosticians tend to generate one or a few hypotheses very early on and thereafter the search for clues is likely to be guided by those hypotheses. With a hypothesis in hand, further information gathering may be constrained, thereby decreasing the likelihood that an alternative hypothesis will be considered and increasing the likelihood of an incorrect diagnosis.

Additionally, once a diagnosis has been made, it is inevitable that the nature of the illness will transform into its idealized form as described by medicine, which catches and tames the disease through language. A disease's mere label has the ability to foster an illusion of control wherein immediately the expert begins to consider the disease as fixed and inert. In today's high-pressure, fast-paced, modern health care environment, where doctors must work efficiently under pressure, it is easy to imagine that doctors often work mindlessly, using familiar diagnostic constructs and their corresponding courses of treatment. Atul Gawande writes in his book *Complications*, it is instead "an imperfect science, an enterprise of constantly changing knowledge, uncertain information, [and] fallible individuals." Every individual is different, every pathogen is different, and therefore it should necessarily follow that every treatment strategy should be different. Yet, in modern medicine, this is rarely the case; Western medicine is embedded within institutionalized and standardized health care.

When I was an intern in the psychology department at Yale, people walked into the clinic and essentially by doing so labeled themselves as "patients." At the time, I saw them this way as well. When we discussed certain behaviors they considered problems—say, anxiety, difficulty making a decision, guilt—I tended to label what they reported as "abnormal," consistent with my use of the "patient" label. Later, when I encountered exactly the same behavior in my acquaintances—the difficulty making a decision or commitment, feelings of guilt, or fear of failure—it seemed odd to me to see the former as problematic and the latter as normal. I became interested in the way labels act as a lens and lead us to see and evaluate that which is seen, while at the same time leading us to ignore what might very well lead to a different evaluation. During that time at Yale, psychologist Robert Abelson and I conducted a study to test this effect.[3] We made a videotape of a rather ordinary-looking man being interviewed about work. For half of the clinicians to whom we showed the tape, we labeled the man being interviewed a "patient." For the other half we labeled him a "job applicant," thus priming a different view of him. We showed the tape to Freudian therapists and behavior therapists. (Behavior therapists are trained to look past labels.) When the man was labeled a "job applicant," both groups saw him as well adjusted. But the Freudians who thought they watched a "patient" saw him as poorly adjusted and in need of therapy. The behavior therapists saw "the patient" as well adjusted.

Labels lead us to go on hypothesis-confirming data searches. That is, we look for evidence to support the label. Since most information is ambiguous, the result is "seek and ye shall find." The label "patient" leads us to examine behavior and life circumstances through a problem-finding lens. The label "patient" also leads us and doctors to search for illness-related symptoms. In both cases, behavior and sensations that could have been seen as typical fluctuations from the norm are interpreted as unhealthy. Moreover, independent cues of health may be totally ignored. The remedy here is actually rather simple. If we entertain the competing hypotheses "We are healthy" and "We are sick" and then go on hypothesis-confirming data searches, we will confirm them both with the result of a more accurate picture of how we are. We will have evidence that we are okay and perhaps also find evidence that we are not. We might see ourselves as generally healthy with a few nagging discomforts, or see ourselves as achy and uncomfortable chronically. Moreover, we might label what we find differently. A sensation that is taken to be an indication of a grave illness is likely to feel worse than one viewed on its own.

Psychologist Dave Rosenhan once conducted a startling study where he and his graduate students attempted to gain admission at a mental health hospital.[4] Using pseudonyms, they arrived at the hospital complaining of hearing voices, auditory hallucinations being a hallmark of schizophrenia. In all other respects, they gave an accurate account of their lives, their relationships, and their experiences. After they had been admitted, they stopped complaining of hearing voices and tried to convince the staff that they ought to be released. It took from seven to fifty-four days, on average nineteen, for them to gain release. The staff discharged them with the diagnosis of schizophrenia in remission, although visitors to the ward reported that they had observed no psychological problems in the students' behavior and other patients suspected that many were not patients at all.

Diagnosis and *prognosis* are words that carry special meaning for us. Patients ask, "What is the diagnosis?" or "What is the prognosis?" almost as if there were no people involved in formulating the answer. Of course, there are, and neglecting that fact greatly alters the effect of the answers. Compare the effect on a patient who hears "your prognosis is bad" with "According to this doctor, based on what he learned in medical school, your prognosis is bad."

If our language were more attuned to the situation, I believe we would take more control over our health. We would be aware that medical facts are not handed down from the heavens, but in fact are determined by people under changing, different conditions. I don't think I can say often enough that medical decisions rest on uncertainty—if there were no uncertainty, there would be no decision to be made. To reveal at least some of this uncertainty would mean that while our doctors may be knowing and caring, they cannot be all-knowing. They are subject to the same biases and value-based judgments as the rest of us. But doctors often feel they have to hide their uncertainty. In extreme cases, they still tend to "hang crepe" (referring to the black crepe hung at funerals): give the worst-case scenario, because if you say the patient will die and the patient lives, everyone is happy, but if you say the patient will be okay and the patient dies, lawsuits may follow.

In some sense, to label a person "terminal" may be the medical world's most egregious error. Hank Williams sang, "No matter how I struggle and strive, I'm never gonna leave this world alive." But the label "terminal" is used to predict premature demise. As we know, doctors can't know when we will die and to tell us we're "terminal" may be a self-fulfilling prophecy. There are no records of how often doctors have been correct or not after making this prediction.

Numbers

The medical profession has a habit of describing people through numbers. We have a blood pressure reading and quantifiable pulse; we can undergo an EKG or an EEG and get more numbers to describe our relative health. Blood work gives us more numbers still. This is efficient in many respects, but the point to be made here is that, like labels, numbers hide ambiguity. Numbers lead us to become people with high or low levels of cholesterol rather than people who are sad or happy, tired or energetic. We become our numbers and behave accordingly, not infrequently making them self-fulfilling prophecies. When I ask the audience in my lectures if they know their cholesterol levels, as I described earlier, those who answer have let their last reading create a very strong illusion of stability; they hold it still, although if asked they would say it is subject to ongoing, natural fluctuations. Their last level has such a strong hold on them that, despite the fact that I have just spoken at length about mindlessly confusing the stability of our mindsets with the stability of the underlying phenomenon, the demonstration never fails. Numbers can not only hide ambiguity but also objectify us, lead to self-fulfilling prophecies. Surely we are more than our health-related numbers.

Numbers also create the illusion of precision. Consider someone who is forty-two years old and someone who is fifty-four years old. What do we know about these two, other than the fact that the first person is younger? Do we know for sure if she's healthier, more energetic, or more creative? Of course not. We know very little no matter what our reason for inquiring about their age in the first place.

Numbers exist along a single continuum and don't convey as much information as we are led to believe. If a person has twice the number of cancer cells as another, what can we predict from just that information? Who will be sicker or die sooner? If the first person was very healthy to start and the latter very sickly, what would you predict?

Body mass index has become a very popular way to measure whether we are overweight. To calculate it, we divide our weight by the square of our height and then multiply by 703. It seems so precise. The only problem is that BMI was never meant to measure an individual's obesity; it was really meant as a general measure of classifying individuals' levels of physical activity. It doesn't differentiate between muscle and fat, so for people with high muscle mass it isn't particularly valid.

Numbers allow for social comparisons. If I have twenty apples and you have thirty apples, you have more. But what does this mean? Each of my twenty apples may be larger than any of yours, and so I have more apple. Yours may be riper, which could make them tastier or over the hill. The numbers don't tell us important information we need to have to more accurately compare.

Researchers have developed a mathematical formula to predict a woman's risk of osteoporotic fracture. The equation has proved 75 percent accurate and will allow physicians to tailor their treatment strategies to help women prevent fractures of fragile bones. While this may seem a great advance, the problem is that we don't know if we are part of the 75 percent or the remaining 25 percent that the formula misses.

Numbers and the tests they represent are not useless. They are tools, and tools can be helpful if used mindfully to guide us and to give us ideas—not to govern what we do or do not do. But they only imperfectly predict our future health and thus should not determine who or how we are.

That Which Is Unspoken

Imagine that you just got your hair cut and a friend remarks, "Oh, you got a haircut." Pause. "I like it." Her pause makes you feel uncertain or even bad, but you find it hard to comment. After all, she did say she liked it.

The meaning of her remark was in the silence, not the words. And the silence was deafening. Likewise, the effects of silence exist in the realm of our health. Imagine that you're eighty years old, visiting the hospital with your adult child. You speak to the physician and she responds to your child instead of to you. The message is clear: you're incapable. You're next visited by two physicians who examine you and then discuss your case with each other, leaving you out of the conversation. You're objectified, and the absence of communication with you reinforces the idea that you are your disease.

Patients often cite the manner in which doctors speak to them as central to their decision to initiate malpractice suits. Researchers Nalini Ambady, Debi LaPlante, Thai Nguyen, Robert Rosenthal, Nigel Chaumeton, and Wendy Levinson looked at the effects of tone of voice in a medical context.[5] The decision to sue a physician is no doubt a difficult one. Research suggests that part of the basis of lawsuits is complaints about interpersonal aspects of care. These researchers investigated whether the surgeons' tone of voice was related to their malpractice claims history. They took brief clips from doctor/patient interactions during office visits, removed the content so that all that was left was tone of voice, and had them coded for attributes such as warmth, hostility, dominance, and anxiety by people who were unaware of the study's hypotheses for warmth, hostility, dominance, and anxiety. They then examined whether there was a relationship between these factors and the physician's malpractice history. When the surgeons' tone of voice was judged to be not friendly and signaled dominance, they were likely to have more claims filed against them. We react to silence, tone of voice, and nonverbal cues even if we are not aware of it.

In research I conducted with my students we were interested in seeing what would happen if an "expert" nonverbally conveys confidence in the face of verbal uncertainty.[6] To look at this, we directed instructors to be confident or unconfident, which was defined here as erect posture (or not), frequent eye contact (or not), and smooth speech (or not). They were then asked to give a sealed envelope to a friend or family member in which a relaxation technique was described in either conditional or unconditional language. The envelopes were sealed so that the instructor couldn't bias the results since he wouldn't know whether the person was in the mindful (conditional) group or the mindless (absolute) group. The friends and family members were told to open and read the contents of their envelopes. When the experiment appeared to be over, the instructor announced that he had a pain in his neck and asked the friend or family member what he should do about it. The major measure we were interested in was whether the person considered the information included in the relaxation technique in their response even though the technique had not mentioned the neck. More than twice as many people in the confident but uncertain group thought to use the information creatively.

What can we do in the face of a culture that quantifies virtually everything? We can remind ourselves what these words and numbers really do and do not tell us. And we can reassert the uncertainty that they hide. More than twenty-five years ago I collected data that I never got around to publishing that are relevant here. I asked elderly adults to participate in a study on language, pronouns in particular. One group was asked to increase the number of times they said "I" over a given week. Control groups increased the number of times they said "me," "he," or "she." At the end of the week we then gave a brief questionnaire asking them how active they were and how much control they felt they had over their lives. The findings revealed that increasing the use of "I" led to an increase in perceived control and activity in this group. While language can subtly lead us to behave, think, and feel in ways not to our advantage, we also can intentionally choose our language to help us go in the direction in which we want to go.

CHAPTER 8

Limiting Experts

Perform all [these duties] calmly and adroitly, concealing most things from the patient while you are attending to him. Give necessary orders with cheerfulness and serenity, turning his attention away from what is being done to him; sometimes reprove sharply and emphatically, and sometimes comfort with solicitude and attention, revealing nothing of the patient's future or present condition.

—The Hippocratic Oath

Human health is a complex issue and stories of medical errors are rampant. Amy Edmondson, who studies patient safety issues in hospitals, has done important research into how medical errors occur, especially in how the medical system facilitates them.[1] Her research makes clear that health care organizations rarely learn from their mistakes, as people are often hesitant to report mistakes, observations, and concerns. Nurses are not infrequently afraid that if they speak up, they will be reprimanded. Not surprisingly, they don't often speak up. Most hospitals, indeed most organizations, prefer to have on their staff "adaptive conformers," people who easily adjust without raising objections and seamlessly correct the errors of others. They make things smoother, unlike the "disruptive questioner," who speaks up when there's a problem, is vocal about the mistakes they and others make, and asks those annoying "Why do we do it this way?" types of questions. The problem, as Edmonson points out, is that organizations that learn—and improve—need the disruptive questioner.

Even small groups are vulnerable to "groupthink," or mindlessness. As psychologist Irving Janis pointed out in his seminal book on the topic, *Victims of Groupthink,* legitimizing the role of a contrarian in a group helps keep the group from mindless conformity.[2] Few hospitals, however, train their staff to avoid mindlessness and to be open to learning from mistakes. While patients are not made part of the safety process, we, as patients, can and perhaps should play the part of the disruptive questioner, as mindful learners about our own health.

The introduction of new technology is especially difficult for group process, especially when it interferes with routine ways of doing things. The surgeon, the nurses, the anesthesiologist, and the perfusionist (a technician who runs the heart-lung bypass machine) all work together in open-heart surgery, and they have done so hundreds of times. Bring in a new piece of equipment and they must now do something different, and that change can be hard. Edmondson found that when new technology for cardiac surgery was introduced, those medical teams with leaders who minimized concern for status differences—in other words, were willing implicitly to admit they didn't have all the answers and take advice from underlings—had the most effective communication, learned the most, and found the transition the easiest.[3]

Would that was more frequently the way of doctor-staff interactions. Instead—and largely because of the institutionalized denial of mistakes that they might otherwise learn from— physician mistakes are so abundant that doctors even have a field of inquiry devoted to their study, iatrogenic medicine—literally, physician-induced disease. According to the Institute of Medicine's 2000 report "To Err Is Human," more people die in American hospitals from medical errors than die nationwide from better-known causes, including highway accidents, breast cancer, or AIDS—up to ninety-eight thousand deaths annually in the United States.[4] Given that physicians are generally caring, intelligent, and well-educated people, how could this be? A close analysis would probably reveal mindlessness as a major culprit. Trained physicians may expect to notice deviations from the norm because of their experience, yet it may be that very experience that blinds some of them. I have wondered what might happen if hospitals teamed up novices and experts. They do that now, of course, but the novices are supposed to learn from the experts and not the other way around. In my scheme, the learning would be mutual. They would be taught to respect that an expert may see what only her training can show her and the novice might notice what the expert was trained to miss.

In *Complications*, Gawande describes a study by researchers Hans Ohlin, Ralf Rittner, and Lars Edenbrandt in which they tested a top cardiologist, who typically read about 10,000 ECGs a year, against a sophisticated computer program to find out which more successfully read ECG information to predict heart attacks.[5] Each read 2,244 ECGs, half of which were known to be from people who had heart attacks. The computer identified 20 percent more of the cases that had led to heart attacks than the cardiologist did. Computers, it seems do a better job at diagnoses than physicians do.

Gawande is a physician and writes brilliantly about the physician's perspective. As he looks at it, the research ought to lead us to conclude that we need to trust technology. The point for me, though, is that the computer still missed 384 cases. One solution he suggests is that we rely more on machines for diagnoses; another of his suggestions along the same lines is that we teach physicians to act like machines.

Thirty years of my research on mindfulness and mindlessness would take issue with both of these suggestions. In my view, the only time we should practice to the point of mindlessness is when two conditions are both met:

1. We have found the best way of doing something.
2. Things don't change.

We know, however, that we can never be sure of the former and the latter is simply never true. It doesn't matter what behavior we want to make "automatic." In matters of our health, since none of us is "us," the statistical mean, there is no best way. And we know that our health is always changing.

Consider, as physicians David Bates and Lucian Leape have, the number of steps involved with prescribing and administering drugs in a hospital setting that can and do go awry:[6]

1. The physician writes the prescription.
2. The prescription is delivered to the secretary.
3. The order is transcribed.
4. The nurse picks up the prescription.
5. The nurse verifies the prescription and transcribes it again.
6. The prescription is given to the pharmacist.
7. The pharmacist dispenses the medication.
8. The medication is given to the nurse.

9. The drug is administered to the patient.
10. The patient receives the drug.

At each step errors are made every day. The average hospital patient receives ten to twenty doses of medication per day and stays for about five days, all of which considerably increases the chances of an error.

To illustrate how even the latter parts of this process can go awry, consider a case the social psychologist Robert Cialdini has written about.[7] A doctor's order for the medication to treat an earache read "administer in Rear." The nurse read it as "rear" instead of "right ear," and inserted the drug in the patient's rectum. The doctor and the nurse were not incompetent; they were mindless.

Even when physicians aren't making obvious errors, problems may arise. While getting a second opinion may seem straightforward, a closer look reveals that the process is not so simple. There are hidden effects of language priming at work here. The word *second* is typically not as good as *first*, regardless of what it modifies. Next, if we take the word of our doctor as truth, then what might we expect when we compare "truth" with an "opinion"? Just as second is less than first, opinion is less trustworthy than fact. In a class demonstration I asked half of my students the following: "A doctor tells you that you need surgery. You get a second opinion and that doctor tells you that you don't need surgery. On an eleven-point scale ranging from zero, meaning 'definitely not,' to ten, meaning 'definitely yes,' how likely are you to get surgery?"

I asked the other half of the students, "A doctor tells you that you need surgery. Another doctor says you don't need surgery. How likely are you to get surgery?" Thus, for the first group a second opinion was mentioned, but not for the second group. When a doctor gave a "second opinion" the average score was 5.

The average response for the group where "second opinion" was not mentioned was 2.5. That is, it became twice as likely that the first doctor's view would be followed when posed against a "second" "opinion."

Dr. John Glick of the Abramson Cancer Center at the University of Pennsylvania has estimated that when patients come to him for second opinions regarding a treatment plan, his view only completely agrees with the first opinion around 30 percent of the time. In another 30 to 40 percent of the cases, he and his colleagues recommend significant changes to the plan. Sometimes his team comes to a completely different diagnosis.[8]

If physicians are all trained in the same approach, they very well may suggest the same course of action; if they are trained differently, different opinions might prevail. Thus, we could have the same people viewing the same facts but differing in their views of them; also, we could have different facts considered by the different physicians. People often don't get second opinions. Is that sensible? If we got a second opinion, regardless of what the next doctor says, it really doesn't tell us what the next fifty doctors would say. It is a very small sample size and as such may not be reliable. On the other hand, there could be a hidden positive side effect. By us—patient and doctor—considering the need for a second opinion, we are implicitly acknowledging uncertainty.

Becoming a Health Learner

To keep our bodies in tune, we usually visit the doctor for an annual checkup and have whatever tests are recommended at that time. If the tests say we are okay, we assume our health is in order and we go forward until next year, unless something out of the ordinary occurs. We often treat our bodies the way we treat our cars, giving over control to the doctor the way we turn our cars over to our mechanic. Once the car passes the inspection or whatever it was treated for, we drive away presuming all is fine. I believe, however, that many of us may be more attentive to our cars than to ourselves. We notice the subtle changes that indicate something is wrong with our cars—a small shimmy, a squealing brake, a muffler that is louder than usual—and we bring the car in for repair (if we can afford it) before the problem gets out of hand even if we know nothing much about cars. We often pay little attention to the subtle changes that our bodies tell us about our health. We've become too reliant on doctors. A useful alternative model may be to use the physician as a consultant. Indeed, perhaps all experts should be called on in this way.[9]

By attending to variability and coming to know our bodies, we are in a better position to have useful information regarding our health. By recognizing the limits to what the physician can know, we can become more confident in the importance of sharing that information. We act as health learners, fully engaged in our health and better able to work with the experts. We become the expert on our individual health and the doctors become our consultants.

If we're our own expert, we might consider using several consultants, not just for different parts of our bodies but to get different views of the same part. Different views signal to us that we are in charge. When we understand the limits of medical data, we can accept that receiving the same view from multiple people does not necessarily mean they are correct. It may only mean that the physicians were trained similarly. We don't become stressed when views differ; we become more aware of how important our own role is to the process. To help us make decisions, we take a more active role not only in considering the information we receive but also in bringing information to the discussion.

We shouldn't wait to be asked questions that our doctor believes are important to help with the diagnosis; doctors' questions are based on normative data, on what is true for most people. If we were the experts, we would offer information that we feel correlates with how we are feeling. Instead of asking "Is this related to that?" we would ask "How might this be related to that?" Doing so encourages a different sort of information search, one that leads our consultants to consider our particular case instead of the general one.

In my seminar on the psychology of decision making, I often ask my students, "Can we prevent conception through nasal spray?" The answer is always no. When I ask, "How could a nasal spray be used to prevent conception?" I get creative answers that recognize that the whole body is connected; those students who are biologically sophisticated search for a possible pathway. Likewise, we should be in charge of at least some of the questions that are considered meaningful to our health.

When we are in charge, we more easily can ask about alternatives without feeling we are challenging the doctor. We might consider asking about other possible medications and their potential side effects as well as alternative treatments, and we should not hesitate to ask about the data on which any of the given advice is based. Once the physician consultant answers these questions, she or he too will become more mindful about the limits of what is known. If we do this in a nonconfrontational way, it is likely to have a humbling affect on the doctor and increase the doctor's willingness to become our consultant and partner in health.

I once gave my seminar students the assignment to investigate health databases and see if they could ask original questions that spoke to any of the health issues we discussed in class. One of my students, Laura Anglin, came up with something provocative that is quite relevant. She examined data obtained from the 1995 Centers for Disease Control Behavioral Risk Factor Surveillance results. Her interest was in health care access and utilization, and she found that of the ten states (Alaska, Arizona, Illinois, Kansas, Louisiana, Mississippi, New Jersey, North Carolina, Oklahoma, and Virginia) that asked the question "Is there one particular health care provider that you usually go to?" the majority of respondents (75 percent to 85 percent) in nine of the states answered "yes." For the tenth state, North Carolina, the opposite was true. Here 65 percent answered that they did not see just one doctor. Elsewhere in the database, she found responses to questions asking how many days per month (from none to thirty) they experienced poor physical and mental health. Compared to the national average, residents in North Carolina were more likely to respond "none" (that is, no days of poor health) than the rest of the country. There were fewer respondents who also were likely to experience poor health for one to two days, three to seven days, and eight to twenty-nine days per month. The results for mental health were the same, with fewer days of poor mental health reported in North Carolina. Like virtually all medical data, these findings are correlations, and by now we all should know that they are meant to be suggestive rather than absolute. That being said, they do support the idea that perhaps seeking the advice of multiple consultants is good for our health.

To seek out several views requires that we become much more involved in the process even if that entails only choosing the people from whom to get the views. Moreover, in being in charge of whom we ask and what we tell them, we prime our own efficacy.

When faced with a diagnosis and the medical options for treatment, the patient is caught in a very difficult dilemma. The impulse to surrender our future treatment wholly to the professional hands of medical practitioners is understandable. Leaving the doctors to make all the choices relieves the existential fear of being responsible for a decision that could in the end hurt us. But not to be involved may hurt us more.

At what point is a patient's cancer considered to be incurable or untreatable? Doctors seem to have to make this judgment call on a somewhat arbitrary basis. As my student Bo Meng pointed out, scientists today cannot even predict the expiration of a carton of milk with total certainty; the temperature at which the carton is stored, the variable conditions of the bacteria that are in the milk, and the degree to which any outside organisms might enter the milk carton are only three of the many factors which influence when the milk will go bad. The sheer complexity of human systems compared to the relative simplicity of a carton of milk ought to suggest that a culture that cannot even determine the course of milk going bad could not possibly have the technology to accurately and precisely determine the threshold at which most cancers cannot be treated.

On the other hand, we ourselves may be able to know. Certainly there are cases in which metastases have reached every point of the body and the patient could die at any minute. But many cases are not so severe even as they are diagnosed as being untreatable and terminal. In such cases, what is the basis of the judgment? To at least some degree, these decisions are arbitrary, and if understanding that would enable the patient to have some reason for hope, she might yet manage to improve her situation. The hope could be based on the awareness of the variability of the experienced symptoms—sometimes it is actually not as bad as at other times. This variability could be communicated to our physician consultant.

While it is true that doctors may know more about cancer than we do, that does not mean that we need to be unaware about the circumstances of our own situation. Today, approximately two-thirds of cancer patients do not actually understand the diagnosis given to them; without understanding the circumstances of diagnosis, dealing with the cancer has to be even more difficult. It would be like trying to play a sport without knowing any of the rules. Yet millions of terminal cancer patients worldwide play this game every day.

Today, we have what is essentially a three-stage continuum for cancer: one can have no cancer, one can have treatable cancer, and one can have terminal or end-stage cancer, which is considered untreatable. Between these categories, however, there are significant distinctions that ought to be made but typically aren't. A patient who is on the line between operable and end-stage cancer, for example, may be deemed inoperable due to a high rate of metastasis or cancer growth. Certain forms of therapy, however, have demonstrated some ability to slow metastatic growth and therefore could conceivably help to bring a patient back into the "treatable" categorization. By asking our physician consultants about the ways in which our disease is different from that of most people in the category, we may come to learn to be more differentiated about our condition.

Given that we know ourselves far better than our medical practitioner will ever be able to, that we can know our unique history and our physical, emotional, and cognitive makeup, we are the ones who will know which treatment options might be best suited to us. Our satisfaction with the treatment will depend on how the particular treatment serves our unique needs, not the needs of some statistically compounded generalized person. Knowing our own values, character, and emotional and cognitive makeup will be essential when making the decision about treatments; keeping these in mind will help us choose according to what would be best for us. So, in the answer to the question of whom to follow if not the doctor, the best answer would be ourselves. After all, while the medical professionals are the best experts on the general course an illness may take, we are the best experts on our particular journey.

CHAPTER 9

Mindful Aging

Old age ain't no place for sissies.

—Bette Davis

For most of us, there is probably no greater time of concern regarding diminished capacity, pain, and disease than late adulthood. Nevertheless, this phase of our lives can still be one of growth. While many of our experienced debilities may be a natural part of aging, many are not and instead are a function of our mindsets about old age. As we saw with the counterclockwise study, even cognitive abilities, vision, and symptoms of arthritis may be improved by becoming more mindful.

Stereotypes regarding the negative consequences of old age are widely known and are almost unconditionally accepted, at least in the West. Studies have shown that older people are seen as forgetful, slow, weak, timid, and set in their ways.[1]

Older adults often hold negative feelings about the elderly that are as strong, if not stronger, than those held by younger adults. In their analysis of studies measuring American's attitudes toward aging, Mary Kite and Blair Johnson found that expressions of negative stereotypes in aging were greatest when people were asked to evaluate the physical attractiveness or mental competence of the elderly.[2] Moreover, research has demonstrated that many of these negative stereotypes about aging are experienced as unconscious or automatic processes.

In addition to their impact on the way older adults are viewed or treated, age-related stereotypes are often internalized by the elderly, and may affect their ability and willingness to engage with younger members of society. Thirty years ago I was part of a small group of doctors and psychologists that came together to examine biology, behavior, and aging. I was the youngest member of the group and the most positive about the aging process. Given that my personal experience with aging was lacking relative to the others, I questioned why this was so. Perhaps the others had already had some firsthand experience with aging or with aging parents that made them more negative about aging. But wasn't it also possible that I had a fundamentally different— not naive—view of aging based on something I too had experienced? Where did I get the idea that aging was not all about decline?

I considered that the word *grandmother* meant "old person" to a young child and that word likely was one of the first introductions many of us have to the idea of being elderly. When I was introduced to the idea of old, my grandmother was reasonably young in age, spirit, and ability. Perhaps my view of old was derived from that experience. Indeed, when we are young, many of us learn what it means to be old from our grandparents and extrapolate from there. If our own grandparents also embraced stereotypes about what it means to be old, we may have inadvertently and unwittingly accepted exaggerated ideas of limits regarding the physical and psychological abilities of the elderly.

More recently I set out to test whether that was indeed the case. My students and I compared elderly subjects who had lived with a grandparent before they were two years old with those who had lived with a grandparent after they were thirteen (as a two-year-old ages to thirteen, of course so too will her grandparent age).[3] For the first group, their grandparents were expected to be and act younger then those of the second group. Given their relative ages, those in the two-year-old group should now, elderly themselves, have a more youthful mindset about old age then the thirteen-year-old group. If that was the case, as the younger group aged they should embrace a "younger" version of old age.

Indeed, we found this to be true. The elderly subjects were independently evaluated by researchers unaware of our hypothesis; those subjects who lived with a grandparent when they were younger and had more youthful mindsets of old age were rated to be more alert. There was also a tendency for them to be more active and more independent. The results suggest that many of us inadvertently may have been taught to grow old by exposure to mindsets that are more limiting than they need be.

There are four lessons from mindfulness research that may be helpful in counteracting the negative effects of stereotypes about the elderly. Based on the research, we need to focus our attention on

1. The criteria used to evaluate the elderly
2. Our inability to see past our own levels of development

3. The concept of change versus decay
4. A more mindful approach to old age, among both the elderly and among those who stereotype them

Let's consider these more carefully.

For young children, the admonition to "act your age" is accompanied by expectations of industry, gravity, and the acceptance of responsibility. For the elderly, however, the idea of acting one's age takes on a more burdensome connotation. Ironically, older people are often expected to act like children, to relinquish a degree of agency, responsibility, and control over their own lives. In its most extreme form, the expectation that adults over a certain age will (or should) begin to "act like old people" can become oppressive, suggesting that behavior is and must be determined by a chronology over which the individual has no control.

Fish can't ride bicycles; therefore, by the criteria established by bicycle riders, fish seem less competent. The difference between the (anthropomorphic) fish here and the elderly lies mainly in how both the elderly and nonelderly view the relationship between an individual and his or her environment. It seems obvious to us that considering their inability to ride a bicycle to be a deficit in fish is ridiculous—the utility of a bicycle should not be judged by its ability to be used by a fish, and the utility of a fish should not be judged by its ability to use an apparatus that was designed for organisms with two arms, two legs, and well-defined bottoms.

Ironically, we often forget this hierarchy of utility when evaluating the competence of the elderly. If an older person has difficulty getting out of a car, for example, we may attribute this difficulty to the weakening of leg muscles and the loss of a sense of balance. Instead, we might consider the inadequacies of a car seat that does not swivel to allow the passenger to emerge straight ahead rather than sideways. While a focus on the inadequacies of automobiles may seem useless, consider how ridiculous it would seem to conclude that a twenty-five-year-old man's difficulty in riding a tricycle is due to an enlargement of his limbs and a loss of flexibility. Tricycles were not made with twenty-five-year-olds in mind; car seats were not made with seventy-five-year-olds in mind. That does not mean, however, that the seventy-five-year-old is deficient when it comes to emerging from cars any more than it means that twenty-five-year-olds are incompetent at tricycle racing.

The old are not the young. Every day, older adults are forced to negotiate an environment that was designed neither by them nor for them. If we were to focus our attention on external reasons for perceived deficits, adapting the bicycle to the fish and not the other way around, we might decrease negative perceptions of the elderly and might encourage creative environmental solutions that benefit people of all ages. Let's again remember the example of the shelf outside an apartment door as a solution for the woman who couldn't manage to carry groceries and open her door at the same time.

Similarly, an elderly adult's mental capacities are often evaluated as if their desires, intentions, and interests were equivalent to those of younger people. To return to fish, it may also seem readily apparent to us that fish don't care much about bikes. However, such an analogy is rarely used to explain (or understand) the behavior of the elderly adult. When a child's parents cannot tell different cartoon characters apart or are unable to identify a top-forties hit from its opening bars, the children do not conclude that their parents have lost either their ability to recognize faces or their memory for music. Rather, they conclude (correctly) that their parents don't care about Pokémon or Britney Spears. It is possible that older adults appear more forgetful simply because they do not care about the same things that younger people care about, including performance on memory tests. If an individual is told a piece of information and does not particularly care about remembering it, he or she may not encode that information in memory. If the person is later asked a question about the information and cannot answer it, has the information been forgotten? Information has to be learned in the first place before it later can be forgotten. Perhaps the elderly are not as forgetful as we assume; they may, in part, simply be more selective encoders.

Researchers who study memory typically find that the young outperform the old. Let's look closely at memory experiments. The experimenter chooses the words the subject is supposed to remember. But all words are not equally familiar to everyone. To make the point, let me take an extreme case. If the list consists of terms such as *Game Boy*, of course the young will outperform the old. If the list contained words like *mahjong*, the old might just as readily outperform the young. The subjects in many experiments are typically college students whose days are spent in the same academic environment as the experimenter. Now, a researcher might object, saying, "I chose these words from the word frequency list." This has the look of objectivity, yet someone made up that frequency list, and all words spoken or read by all people are hardly equally likely to have been considered. As we discussed earlier, there are hidden decisions and there are hidden deciders. But the "facts," when they reach the public, are presented as if they are immutable truths given to us from the heavens, rather than that they are based on decisions made by people who may have had us in mind and may not have.

Meaningless and Meaningful Remembrances

It is often observed, anecdotally, that older people have intact memories of events that occurred in their childhoods but poor memories for events of the recent past. Perhaps older memories are more meaningful to the elderly; this type of information was worthy of encoding in the past and is worthy of retrieval in the present. When the performance of an older person "falls short" on some measure, we invariably see this as a failure of the individual rather than question the relevance of the measure. And yet we never doubt the competence of the fish. What keeps nonelderly researchers from shifting their attention to the inadequate measure? In a recent study, for example, it was found that older subjects retain the gist of what they read but not the particulars. Given that the subject matter surely was chosen by a younger experimenter, how likely is it that more than just the gist is important for their lives?[4]

I meet many more people now than I did in my youth. I also have more status. In my youth I remembered their names. Now I tend not to. If I meet a person enough times so that it matters, I will learn his name. Am I forgetful, busy, self-involved, tired, bored, all or none of the above?

It is difficult to see past one's own level of development. Ask a child what it would be like to be thirty and he or she will show remarkably little insight. Ask a thirty-year-old what it would be like to be eighty years old and, whether we care to admit it or not, the same thing may happen. Older people are often judged as if they subscribe to the same set of values and reference points as those who judge them. For example, some researchers have suggested that in old age people naturally regress to a state of childhood. There is an important difference, however, between the resumption of behaviors that one exhibited in the past and the enactment of these behaviors for the first time. For example, if both seven-year-old Jimmy and ninety-seven-year-old James tell a dinner guest her stories are boring, they may be using the same words, but they are hardly exhibiting the same behavior. A mindful analysis would suggest that Jimmy is uninhibited, meaning that he has not yet learned the socially appropriate response to dinner conversation. In contrast, James is disinhibited. He is well aware of the norms of social behavior but has chosen to ignore them. The observed similarity in the two behaviors creates a false equation of old age with childhood.

Not being able to see past one's own level of development, coupled with a tendency to understand behaviors in ways that are most relevant to the observer, can lead to a whole range of incorrect, but stereotypically coherent, attributions about the elderly's behavior. Perhaps we would all benefit from considering other reasons to explain why the elderly may exhibit stereotypic (and "negative") behavior. For example, forgetfulness might be seen as a judgment that the information was not worth learning or even positively as the ability to focus intensely on the present. Driving slowly might reflect an accumulated wisdom of the risks involved.

Aging or Decaying?

Aging means change, but change does not mean decay. While the term *development* can be applied to changes over the entire life cycle of a person, the term is commonly taken to refer only to the first two decades of life. The influence of this attitude is persistent. Young people are described as "developing," whereas persons changing in their later years are typically described as "aging." It is like day and night, where *day* might formally refer to the entire twenty-four-hour span but is informally used to refer to the brighter side of day. So, too, *aging* has come to refer to the darker side of development. In this case, however, the nominal distinction has great consequence. To make changes in later life one must fight against all sorts of consensually held preconceptions before they are "recognized" as growth. This struggle for legitimate recognition would be less strenuous if development were cast in other contexts. Right now, our stereotypes about the negative aspects of aging prevail.

For example, an eighty-year-old man is frustrated by the fact that he no longer can play tennis the way he could when he was fifty. But perhaps the problem is not that he can no longer play the same way but that he is still trying to do so. Venus Williams, who is six foot three and has one of the largest grip sizes in women's tennis, and Amanda Coetzer, who is five foot two and has one of the smallest, cannot possibly play with comparable strategies, nor would it occur to them to do so. Coetzer, however, is well aware that her small stature allows her to be quick on the court, and Williams understands that her height gives her stroke tremendous power. Because his social environment and mindless encoding of stereotypes has taught the eighty-year-old tennis player that his game is aging, not developing, it may never occur to him to adapt his game based on the identification of new skills. Because differences between young and old people are taken not as differences but as decrements, we are not likely to find ways that older people might metaphorically "change their game."

If we do begin to notice such potential adaptations, we might still make the mistake of seeing these changes as compensatory: "Since I can't do it that way, I'll do it this way." Instead, we could look for ways in which adaptations might be advantageous to individuals of all ages, we could thus learn from the very people we now feel sorry for.

Chronology aside, our age is relative and may vary depending on the domain in question. Just as we can pay attention to the variability in our symptoms to gain control, we can attend to the variability in our competences. Mary may feel old when playing bridge with her neighbors but young when playing Monopoly with her grandchildren, and even younger when playing the French horn in the community orchestra. As we've seen, certain contexts place labels on older people that then become difficult to escape. The more we are able to see ourselves and each other in a variety of social contexts, taking on a diversity of social roles, the more each may be viewed mindfully.

The relationship between age-related changes and physical and mental decline is not a universal truth. Think back to the experiment in which Becca Levy and I studied young and elderly members of two communities that do not hold negative stereotypes of elderly adults—the mainland Chinese and American deaf. The experiment confirmed that elderly in both the mainland Chinese and American deaf cultures outperformed the American hearing elders on four memory tasks. If memory loss in old age were determined only by a biological mechanism of decay, the elderly of these two cultures probably would not be expected to demonstrate better memory skills than the elderly American participants.

The results indicated that age-related changes do not inevitably mean decline and research on memory loss in general bears out this conclusion. Though some researchers have argued that such a decline is inevitable and have documented consistent trends, others believe that some aspects of the deterioration of memory may be environmentally determined, shaped by expectations and social contexts.

Many negative consequences of aging are the result of priming. In one study conducted by Becca Levy and her colleagues, older adults were subliminally primed with either positive or negative aging stereotypes.[5] Stereotype primes in the positive condition were the words *accomplished*, *advise*, *alert*, *astute*, *creative*, *enlightened*, *guidance*, *improving*, *insightful*, *sage*, and *wise*. Stereotype primes in the negative condition were *Alzheimer's*, *confused*, *decline*, *decrepit*, *dementia*, *dependent*, *diseases*, *dying*, *forgets*, *incompetent*, *misplaced*, and *senile*. When asked to take a variety of mathematical and verbal tests, participants exposed to the negative stereotypes experienced a heightened cardiovascular response due to stress, including elevated systolic and diastolic blood pressure and increased heart rate.

Priming, of course, can result in positive changes as well. Priming health and competence could reverse some of the debilitations assumed to be hard-wired in humans. Recall the plant study I discussed at the beginning of the book, in which we gave elderly residents in a nursing home the autonomy to make decisions and responsibility over a plant that resulted in significant differences on measures of alertness, happiness, active participation, and a general sense of well-being just three weeks later. Eighteen months later, these differences had grown to not just measures of physical and psychological health but also mortality rates. In a somewhat similar study, psychologist Richard Schultz found that increasing control by providing institutionalized elderly adults with the opportunity to decide when they would be visited also resulted in improvement on psychological and physical health measures.[6]

Charles Alexander and I, along with colleagues, replicated these results in a later study where both mindfulness as we study it (noticing novelty) and transcendental meditation (predicted to enhance mindfulness after meditation practice) were used to promote mindfulness.[7] Both mindfulness-producing groups showed marked enhancement in intellectual functioning as well as physical health. They also exhibited an increase in perceived control, felt significantly younger, and were rated by nurses as improved on mental health. Further, both groups lived longer than the control group during the three-year follow-up period. All of these findings suggest that creating environments in which the elderly are challenged to counteract stereotypes rather than expected to express them may diminish their negative effects.

Mindless Institutional Living

Most of the retreat participants in the counterclockwise study had been living with their adult children, which meant that the houses they lived in and even their rooms were not fully their own. Given these circumstances, our subjects lacked the household reminders of their youth and their past vigor. The retreat was conceived to provide a better environment for them in that regard. While it was not completely personalized, the rooms were full of magazines of that week from twenty years ago, which would signal a more robust time in their lives. And all of the rooms were different, which was important both as a memory aid and to convey the feeling of living in an inn for the week, rather than an institution. If I lived in a nursing home where each room was the same, I'm sure I'd walk into the wrong room as often as my own. (I don't think this is just true for me, although truth be told I've never understood how those mice my colleagues run in mazes ever find their way out.)

Before the study began, everyone was asked for a recent photo of themselves and one from twenty years ago. We distributed the latter among the experimental group and photos of their present selves to members of the control group. We did this to help the experimental group members recognize each other as younger and more vigorous.

We requested that participants not bring anything more recent than 1959 to the retreat with them. We specifically asked them to bring one small item that they had had since they were young. John brought a pen; Fred brought a beer stein; Ben brought his Zippo lighter, which he had bought right after he saw it used by the cowboy in the old Marlboro commercial. Irving brought a comb and brush set that had belonged to his father. Peter brought his Brooklyn Dodgers cap, and when we commented on it a few days into this exercise, he railed about the Dodgers moving to Los Angeles just a couple of years "earlier." Max hadn't remembered to bring anything, but he seemed to have an unusual attachment to the issue of *Sports Illustrated* that we put in his room. The main living room had multiple copies of *Life* magazine and the *Saturday Evening Post* from that same week in 1959.

Old radio programs—*Gunsmoke* episodes and Bob and Ray routines—played on an old radio, just as they might have in the past. The men seemed to especially like *Ted Mack's Original Amateur Hour*, Milton Berle, Perry Como, and of course Jack Benny. All of these choices in entertainment were meant to bring forth thoughts and emotions of an earlier time.

Probably the most important choice we made regarding physical cues was that nothing was done at the retreat to make it more "elderly-friendly." While for older adults, obstacles are typically removed to make life easier, the lack of obstacles signals incompetence. At the retreat, how to overcome minor difficulties, such as negotiating stairs, getting to their room by themselves, or figuring our how to pick up a dropped item, was left to the men to figure out so that they might enjoy feelings of accomplishment.

When we took our measures, we tried to weave them into the events taking place because we felt that medical equipment and psychological tests in and of themselves often signal problems. For example, we tested memory with a game where we showed slides of noteworthy people and they hit a key as soon as they recognized who it was. The experimental group was quicker and more accurate.

In the information packet we sent out before the trip, everyone was told what kind of clothing to bring. They were told not to bring anything fashionable but instead to bring comfortable and preferably very old clothing. The staff was also given recommendations for their attire. They were told to dress in "timeless" attire, rather than to wear lab coats or anything that could signal a difference in status. Given the clothing that graduate students tend to wear, this posed no hardship. We were all more or less equals with nothing external to signal to the participants that we were in charge, that they were being watched, that they were expected to have problems, etc. We were essentially people interacting with people where our various roles were not made salient. We essentially gave up any external markers of our roles, befriended the participants as individuals instead of as elderly men, and spent the week in an environment that by virtually all accounts seemed timeless.

Currently too many of our parents and grandparents live in institutional settings where mindless routine prevails. Even the decor of some of these places suggests the absence of change. If mindfulness is life-begetting, as several of our experiments suggest, perhaps excessively scheduled lives portend premature death. If finding a way to live mindfully in these environments is difficult and thus unlikely, then what is the alternative to excessive mindlessness? There may be three alternatives: somehow finding a mindful life, premature death, or senility. As odd as that sounds, I'm suggesting that senility may be a mindful response to an overly routinized environment. As described below, our research bears this interpretation out. If senility is a cry for more mindfulness, it may be biologically adaptive even if socially maladaptive.

To examine this, in 1979, psychologists Ronnie Janoff-Bulman, Pearl Beck, Lynn Spitzer, and I compared people in nursing homes who had been labeled "senile" with those who were not so labeled.[8] We held disease constant. Thus, a person might have heart disease with or without a diagnosis of senility. We found those labeled senile actually lived six to nine years longer. This study on senility was conducted before brain scans became popular, and so those people today whose brain scans reveal dementia may be exhibiting something different from our subjects—we don't know. Still, many people even today, especially those away from large medical complexes, are diagnosed from small samples of their behavior and, like those we described, may be seeking a mindful alternative to the environments they are experiencing.

If the old are expected to decline physically, it is unlikely that they will be given the extra medical attention that could make a difference. Moreover, small improvements are not likely to be noticed, and they will be the first to be denied help when medical resources are in short supply. The problem is exacerbated by older adults accepting this stereotype to be true. Neither the medical community nor the elderly patients themselves question the unconditional nature of their assumptions. Even worse, adult children often feel helpless in dealing with their aged parents. Perhaps instead we could start questioning all of these mindsets.

Mindlessly Giving In to Negative Stereotypes

The unconscious enactment of negative stereotypes is linked to three other processes that can lead to negative health outcomes among older adults. The first process is a self-fulfilling prophecy of decline. To the extent that older adults expect aging to be associated with physical or cognitive detriments, these expectations may be confirmed through conscious pressures on behavior. Another aspect of such a self-fulfilling prophecy relates to the interpretation of ambiguous information. Because they expect to experience deficits, older adults may be more likely to interpret their own behavior and experience as evidence of their physical decline. Consider a situation in which an older man spends the day working with his granddaughter in the garden and wakes up the next morning with a sore back. Because he knows that older people are likely to have aches and pains, he attributes his sore back to his advanced age. This association—"My back hurts; it must be because I'm old"—can act as a self-generated prime, causing the grandfather to walk more slowly than the sore back would dictate, which, in turn, confirms additional age-related stereotypes. Because of the grandfather's association of age and physical decline, it never occurs to him to discover that his granddaughter awoke with an equally sore back, which she attributed to four hours of weeding.

An individual's negative expectations about aging can also interact with the expectations of others, creating an interactionally fulfilling prophecy. Imagine that both George (age eighty-three) and Martha (age forty-five) believe that aging is associated with cognitive decline. When Martha tries to explain a concept to George, she attempts to simplify her explanation, but this oversimplification leaves out certain details. George notices the simplified way in which Martha is speaking, and her omission of certain details leaves him confused. Research suggests that not only will George worry that his confusion is a result of his age (rather than attribute it to a deficiency in Martha's explanation), but his behavior will change to confirm the expectations of both conversation partners. In a positive example of this, research has demonstrated that students whose teachers were told that they were on the verge of an intellectual growth spurt not only were more likely than their peers to be evaluated more favorably by their teachers but also exhibited actual increases in IQ compared with students assigned to a control group.[9] Many investigations of self-fulfilling prophecies have demonstrated similar effects on the attitudes and behavior of both partners in a given interaction.

Feelings of dependence also have been directly linked to negative health effects. Negative stereotypes about aging may increase psychosocial vulnerability to health risks among the elderly by exacerbating a loss of control. Research demonstrates that it is often not the exercise of control that is important but rather the belief (be it true or not) of one's ability to exercise control in a given situation. If environmental constraints or physical limitations deny individuals the opportunity to exercise control, we may experience the type of "learned helplessness," in which we continue to abdicate control once environmental constraints are no longer present, that we saw in Martin Seligman's helplessness experiments. This loss translates directly into the absence of the exercise of control in health care settings; individuals over sixty often report that they desire less control over health-related decisions, preferring less information and asking health care professionals to make decisions for them. Research, however, has demonstrated that the relationship between age and decreased desire for control is mediated by perceived self-efficacy. That is, individuals who perceive themselves to be less able to make decisions report less desire for control.[10]

To the extent that physical or environmental changes limit control for older adults, the perception of control over some aspects of life becomes even more important. In a study by psychologists Lawrence Perlmuter and Angela Eads, older adult males who sought assistance from a memory clinic were presented with a memory test in which they were either given a degree of control over the task or given no control.[11] Subjects in the enhanced-control condition showed improved performance on the test compared to subjects in the no-control condition. In a second study, these improvements extended to subsequent memory tasks, suggesting that increased control may motivate performance in the same way that loss of control impedes it.

The third mechanism through which the negative stereotypes of aging may hurt older adults is through the very institutions created to ensure their care. Health care professionals are not immune to the impact of negative stereotypes about aging and may be subject to biases that increase health risks for older individuals. Nurses make more negative attributions about older adults than any other age group, and misconceptions about older adults and their concerns have been identified as barriers to providing health care by health care professionals. Similarly, physicians have been observed to offer less aggressive treatment to older patients without considering other medical factors that might affect the treatment's success or the course of the illness.

In a survey of adults over fifty in the United States and Canada, more than 50 percent of respondents reported instances in which their health care provider attributed an ailment simply to their age or told them that they were "too old" to engage in an activity.[12] In these ways, negative stereotypes about older adults have the potential to directly affect health outcomes by limiting access to medical care, disrupting patient-provider communication, and reducing treatment options.

Many of the care systems created to provide treatment for older adults perpetuate feelings of dependence and loss of control. Research conducted in nursing homes suggests that "over-helping" can lead individuals to infer their own helplessness and incompetence, causing them to do poorly at a task that they had previously been able to accomplish. (This is what the counter-clockwise study showed as well.) A series of research studies conducted by Margret Baltes and colleagues demonstrated that a "dependence support script" defines many social interactions between older adults and social partners, such that dependent behavior is reinforced through helping while independent behaviors are ignored.[13] These studies demonstrate that dependence support scripts are more pronounced and prevalent in institutional settings. Interestingly, the behavioral particulars need not change to effect a reversal of these effects. Consider a nursing home program, for example, that has children "adopt a grandparent" versus one that has a program in which elders "adopt a grandchild." In the latter, the elder is implicitly in control.

Behavioral Monitoring

Years ago, psychologist Lawrence Perlmuter and I developed a technique to enhance control for nursing home residents that foreshadowed the idea of increasing control through attention to variability. Briefly, we had residents focus their attention on the alternatives they rejected even for their most mundane activities, such as what kind of juice to have for breakfast. This monitoring task served to remind them of the choices implicit even in the most mindless routine activities, and increased their perceived control accordingly.

For many older adults, aging may be associated with a narrowing of self-definition. Changes in ability, opportunity, or perspective may cause older adults to focus on their current restrictions, comparing themselves with what they "used to do." An understanding of aging as a process of increasing limitation or loss may result from equating behavior with identity—that is, defining an aspect of self in terms of only a limited and specific set of activities. For example, imagine an older adult with a strong identity as a painter who develops arthritis in his hands to an extent that makes it difficult for him to hold a brush. A mindless assessment of this situation might result in encouraging this individual to come to terms with the fact that at some point he may no longer be able to be a painter. He might be assisted in developing a new hobby, or asked to reflect on all the wonderful art he produced in his youth. Instead of coming to terms with the end of his career as a painter, this individual might be encouraged to reconsider the way he paints—holding the brush in his teeth or experimenting with finger painting, spray cans, or spilling paint on the canvas. But even if this individual is not interested in or satisfied with these modifications to his painting style, a mindful reconsideration of his abilities would focus on broadening the concept of "painter" to include a host of activities in which the individual can still engage and excel. Being "a painter" can mean a particular way of seeing the world, a way of understanding and interpreting art, a gift for matching color and tone with meaning. This individual does not have to give up those aspects of self, and will always be a painter, even if he is not painting at the moment. More to the point, even if he still paints with a brush, now he will do different things with it than before his arthritis. If he notices the differences as differences, not decrements, he may develop an entirely new way of painting for himself. Broadening both our understanding of identity-defining categories and the variety of environmental and motivational influences that shape behavior may allow older individuals to focus on continuity across the life span, rather than loss.

Similarly, older adults can consider themselves athletes long after their physical stamina or agility may prevent them from engaging in their preferred sport, like our older tennis player above. This idea of concept broadening stands in contrast to recommendations of downward social comparison, in which older adults are encouraged to feel good about themselves as "an athlete" because they are still in excellent shape compared to people of their own age. In contrast, this framing of self-definition does not rely on social comparison, and for that reason is both more satisfying and more enduring.

Increasing Discrimination

A mindful approach to the world may reduce prejudice and stereotyping by increasing discrimination not against people but between them. Mindfulness through active distinction making about given individuals prevents one characteristic from dominating or defining them. As such, global characteristics such as "Tom and Joan are old" might become more differentiated and may be perceived as specific attributes of an individual rather than a class of persons: "Tom has gray hair and whistles; Joan wears red nail polish and walks with a cane." Without this differentiation, for example, the correlation between apparent age and chronological age is likely to be exaggerated as a result of illusory correlation. Consider the fact that while older people are more likely to have gray hair than younger people, we can all think of exceptions. However, the strangers we see every day are typically taken as confirmation of this hypothesis; young people with gray hair are assumed to be chronically older than they are, and old people with darker hair are assumed to be younger. So the correlation may not be nearly as high as we presume.

The same would be true, of course, for characteristics and abilities. By increasing the distinctions we notice about individuals in the world around us, we may improve our ability to discriminate among them and sharpen our understanding of the futility of arbitrary categorizations.

This is important in its own right but also because cognitive decline typically leads to physical decline. The assumption of cognitive decline, as we've said, overlooks several factors:

1. Old and young are motivated by different things.
2. The tests of cognitive ability have all been designed by younger adults. Consider again the results of a memory test using words such as *Game Boy* versus one using *mahjong*.
3. Is it that the older we get, the harder it is to remember facts, or is it that instances of a rule matter less once one has the general rule?
4. Our attention to interpersonal concerns can masquerade for cognitive loss and may be an asset and not a liability (who cares who did it or why; life starts right now). "For-

getting" harsh interactions allows us to go forward without dwelling on the past; forgetting is a cue to be in the present.

Older adults may face real difficulties associated with aging. Both the elderly and the not yet elderly, however, might be better off by questioning the applicability of age-sensitive measures of competence; by realizing that one can't see past one's own level of development; by accepting that aging means change, but not necessarily decay; and by promoting autonomy, active distinction making, and attention to variability for ourselves and those around us.

Seeing "Them" Differently

Our bodies are constantly changing, a statement that if mindfully accepted may allow us to gain control of functioning that appears only to be diminishing to the mindless observer. And each of our parts, so to speak, is changing at a different rate and in a different way. In the same way, our culture is made up of people who are aging differently. There is a tendency to see any group as a single entity—they all look the same and act the same. Hence for the not-yet-old, seniors may seem more similar to one another than a closer look would reveal. We notice differences among in-group members because of more interaction with them and greater need for their individuation. It would behoove us, however, to turn our mindfulness to the older adults we see around us. Just as we might ask "Why today at this time does my asthma seem better?" we could be asking "Why at this time does John at ninety-three or Nancy at ninety-six seem so healthy?" We can attribute their active minds and bodies to genetic factors, but to do so denies the possibility of learning from them. We can assume they spent their younger lives exercising and eating healthfully, but that provides little that would be helpful to us if we are over fifty ourselves. What are they doing right now? The more specific we are in our attributions for their strengths, the easier it is to learn from them. Although we can never know if our understanding is correct, we still gain in at least three ways: our observations increase our mindfulness, our mindful noticing is likely to be positively experienced by them, and the changes we make for ourselves may be good for us even if our understanding of them was wrong. For example, if I notice that Nancy walks in the morning before she eats a large breakfast and I assume that this may be the reason for her good health and so I decide to try it, I may benefit even if her good health is primarily the result of genetics.

If everyone in the family was taught to be mindful, problems for all of us could diminish. When my grandmother was diagnosed as senile many years ago, as I described earlier, I thought it must be wrong since in my presence she was as sharp as ever. When I got a little older I learned that people who are diagnosed with senility (we now call it dementia) don't show the symptoms all of the time. For a while that settled it for me. For her, like for most people with the diagnosis, the problems manifest often but not all of the time, so I thought the diagnosis might be correct. In the end, they discovered that the senility diagnosis was wrong and that what she had was a brain tumor. I can only return again to the issue of having symptoms some but not all of the time. I think all of us on occasion probably seem irrational to those close to us. How irrational and for how long do we need to be in that state to warrant a diagnosis of dementia? If we are completely "out of it" for 15 percent of the day, would that qualify? Twenty percent? Who decides?

There is now another question that occupies my thoughts. For argument's sake, let's say a person is irrational 65 percent of the time, so most would think there is a real problem. What is happening for the remaining 35 percent of the time? Isn't this what researchers studying the problem should consider? If my grandmother had been senile much of the day but fine when she was with me, was it that supportive and nonthreatening circumstances worked against the disease? Was it the time of day I was visiting? If so, what differentiates her biology at those times from the rest? And so on. From this perspective different questions for examination occur, and with different questions different answers are likely to follow.

My father—the man with the self-described "bad memory"—is, at this writing, in an assisted-living facility in Boca Raton, Florida. I'm actually writing this from his room while he is resting. We finished playing cards. He taught me gin when I was a child, and whenever I visited him since that time, we played.

As we were well into the first game and my hand started looking good, I tried to figure out whether I should let him win or whether that was too condescending. While I was busy making this judgment, he declared that he had gin. I looked at his cards and he indeed won. He won the next game also. I'm on the faculty of one of the world's leading universities and I'm not a bad card player. Nevertheless, this man who is supposed to be suffering from dementia just won three out of five of the games we played.

CHAPTER 10

Becoming Health Learners

*If you are mindful that old age has wisdom for its food, you will so
exert yourself in youth that your old age will not lack sustenance.*

—Leonardo da Vinci

As the end of the counterclockwise study drew near, I couldn't
help but notice the difference in the participants' appearance.
They stood taller, walked faster, and spoke with more confidence. When we took Fred's blood pressure the last morning,
we asked him to raise his shirt sleeve to expose his left arm and he
kindly but assertively said he'd rather we use his right arm. He
knew what was comfortable for him better than we did and
didn't hesitate to tell us. John had come to share my appetite and
seemed to walk to dinner faster and faster each evening. When
Fred told him he shouldn't eat so much or so fast, John replied,

"Who says so?" After a few days, this had become almost a re-frain. When one of the men would tell another what he should or shouldn't do, the response not infrequently was, "Who says so?" Sometimes they smiled when they said it.

When I first wrote about this study in 1981, I hesitated to de-scribe my experience fully, thinking that to do so might taint ac-ceptance of the experimental findings and that the results would be rejected. I am older now and there does not seem much risk in describing what to me were the most rewarding aspects of the entire experience. These were men who many would have thought to be on their last leg before we set out on this adventure. At the end, one of them had begun to walk without using his cane.

On the last day of the retreat, we waited outside for the bus to take us back to Cambridge. One of my graduate students had brought a football to throw around with the other students. I asked Jim, a man who had seemed so frail to me in his interview, if he wanted in on a game of catch. He agreed, and quickly a few of the others drifted over to join us. In just minutes, we were in the midst of an impromptu touch football game on the front lawn. No one would mistake it for the NFL, but at the start of the study no one would have predicted this was possible. Fifteen minutes later, amazed at what just happened, energized, and a little reluctant, I boarded the bus home.

When we returned to the lab in Harvard's William James Hall, we set about analyzing the data we had collected over the course of the study. I didn't yet know if we had chosen the right measures to assess improvement or whether the data would be statistically significant, but in all honesty it really didn't matter that much to me. The two weeks I spent watching these men change—one week with each group—was ample payback for all the effort we went through.

As I've said, we did indeed find improvements for both

groups of participants in measures of their physical strength, manual dexterity, gait, posture, perception, memory, cognition, taste sensitivity, hearing, and vision. The group for whom we turned the clock back (those who experienced 1959 as the "present"), however, showed greater improvements on most of the measures. In order to confirm our sense that the men seemed to be healthier and more youthful, we had four people who knew nothing about the study view random photographs of the men taken both before they left for the retreat and on the last day. These are the objective observers I briefly mentioned earlier. Each of them were shown either the before or the after photo of the person, but not both, and we asked them to judge the age of the men. They rated the appearance of the participants for whom we turned the clock back as being more than two years younger at the end of the study than they were at the start.

These improvements were the result of one week spent with a group of strangers. Imagine the possibilities if our culture afforded us a different set of mindsets than we have about old age.

We Can Influence Our Lives if Not Our Deaths

While death may be inevitable and life after death unknowable, we certainly can influence life before death. If we put together all that we have learned thus far, we come up with a new way to understand health. Several of the research findings I've presented provide reasons to question the traditional way we respond to medical information and the motivation to find a new way. When we recognize that doctors can only know so much, that medical data are not absolute truths, that language hides decisions that rob us of choice, that incurable really means indeterminate, and that our beliefs and most of the relevant external world are social constructions, we should be ready to seek a new way. If we attend to variability and understand that there are always small improvements we can make, we are ready to embark on this new path.

When I first hear my car's brakes screech, I realize the brake pads need to be changed. I could, however, be more attuned to them on a daily basis, so that I recognize there is a problem after hearing a slightly less obvious and aversive noise. I could next become more attuned, so that I catch the problem even sooner, and eventually I could be so sensitive to the workings of my brakes that I avert a problem not yet arisen. The same may be done with respect to our health. If I knew that my ankle felt a bit "funny" I could be more attentive to avoid the possible sprain or break that is just around the corner. If I noticed subtle changes in my skin tone or the color of my urine I could spot trouble soon enough to take action before an emergency situation arises.

But we have to make a decision to be more mindful to accomplish this. I sometimes go full out until I virtually collapse. I often stop eating only after I feel stuffed. Clearly there are signals to which I could attend sooner that would lead me to stop and rest in the first instance and put down my fork in the second.

When I was twentysomething I fainted every so often. The doctors scared me when they suggested that I might have a mild case of epilepsy. When the tests they had ordered were finished, they concluded I didn't have epilepsy, but they didn't know what was wrong with me. I took matters into my own hands and attempted to "catch" myself sooner and sooner each time I felt as though I was about to faint. I'm not sure exactly what I did, but the fainting stopped. Of course, as a scientist, I have to acknowledge the possibility that it might have stopped on its own. That being said, my attempt to control my condition was empowering in its own right.

Oftentimes things feel impossible even though we recognize that they are not. As I pointed out already, if it is overwhelming to think about losing fifty pounds, imagine losing an ounce. When we engage this strategy, we will probably see that our progress doesn't follow a straight line. Sometimes we can easily go forward and sometimes not. Sometimes yesterday's progress is today's failure. This changing aspect of attending to small steps and seeing how unsteady progress may be is perhaps the most important part of pursuing the Reverse Zeno Strategy. The result is attention to variability.

There are practical ways we can use what we've learned about variability across most situations in which we must confront problems. We might consider keeping a diary in which we note for every two- or three-hour block of time whether or not we have experienced a particular symptom and if so, what the surrounding circumstances were. This can accomplish several things. First, it will show that most of the time we probably don't have the symptom. Second, it may reveal some similarity in the circumstances where we do have the symptom and implicitly suggest ways of controlling it. Third, taking the time to notice in order to keep the diary is mindful and has its own advantages. Researcher James Pennebaker has found in his studies that mindful writing results in many health improvements, including fewer stress-related visits to the doctor, improved immune system functioning, reduced blood pressure, improved lung function, improved liver function, fewer days in the hospital, improved mood and affect, a feeling of greater psychological well-being, and reduced depressive symptoms before examinations, to name a few of his findings.[1]

Many of us are blind to the changes in our bodies and simply wait to fall apart. That's what my friend Mary did. Mary was told she had a lump in her breast and needed a biopsy. Not surprisingly, she was scared. At first I tried to reassure her with the statistics regarding women of her age. The numbers suggested that she was an unlikely candidate for cancer. She rejected that argument because she knew that even if the odds were low, she could be the one in a hundred. I told her, "No worry before its time"; if it turned out to be cancer, there would be plenty of time to worry if she needed to. The biopsy could not be scheduled immediately, however, so she had to live in fear. Her story turned out fine; the tumor was benign. What would have helped her during that difficult time while she waited for her answer? Given that our belief that cancer is a death sentence is so strong and our psychological strength when afraid so weak, most reasoning will fall on deaf ears. What if she considered how she could help herself right then? If she paid attention to the variability in her body's physiological state—sometimes better and sometimes worse—and thought about how she might use diet, exercise, or other factors to improve it, she could begin to feel back in control and thus improve her psychological state. Simply attempting to help ourselves can turn out to be an invaluable way to do so. Waiting was hard and so we shouldn't wait. Distraction may be useful but often doesn't last very long. In Mary's case, the "distraction" was actually attention to the problem. If we are taking care of ourselves in this way, we do not seem as helpless to others and, more important, to ourselves.

Recent research tells us that dogs are able to discern if someone has a tumor.[2] If we enhance our ability to sense subtleties, eventually we may be able to do so as well—one very small step at a time. The fact that we can't do it now only means that we haven't yet found the way. We are more likely to find the way, however, if we at least are open to the possibility.

Mindfulness, as I've studied it for more than thirty years, is the simple process of actively drawing distinctions. It is finding something new in what we may think we already know. It doesn't matter what we notice—whether it is smart or silly. Simply noticing is what is important. When we do this, we will find ourselves in the present, more aware of context and perspective and ready to take advantage of opportunities that would otherwise go unnoticed. My social psychology colleagues are fond of saying that behavior is context-dependent. I am saying that if we are mindful, we can create the context.[3]

We can wait for science to catch up and then do as it suggests, or we can begin today to become more involved in our own care. The problem is that scientists often fall into the same mindless trap as the rest of us, and so the wait may be quite some time. Consider the following of how our categories trap us once we forget that they were initially based on decisions with uncertainty. As scientists, we divide the brain in half and compare the right and left hemispheres. This works in many respects, but it also limits us when we forget that other ways of categorizing the brain could also work. Right now we study the brain by looking at the right or the left hemispheres because the hemispheres are clearly demarcated in space and are anatomically similar. If we focus on the right side of the brain and a problem occurs there, for example, we might conclude that treatment would be hopeless since all of that part of the brain is not functioning. If, on the other hand, we divided the brain into top and bottom, rather than right and left, for argument's sake, we might see that some of the brain still functions, which might provide the motivation to figure out how to recruit that part in "fixing" the rest.

Right now we wait for the medical world to dole out medication that has been tested against a placebo. Others have acknowledged that the placebo itself is powerful medication. In many of the studies illustrating the placebo effect, subjects were deceived into thinking that the pill they were taking was "real" medication, that the coffee they were drinking was caffeinated, or that the leaves they were touching were real poison ivy. In all of these examples of the power of the placebo, the question remains: who is doing the healing? Since the placebo is inert, we must be the ones responsible for the improvement. If we are responsible for the placebo's effectiveness, we should be able to learn a more direct way to affect our health—we can ask, "Given that this pill is not doing anything but priming our thoughts to be healthy, why do we need a pill at all?" We should also ask if the placebo effect in part can be attributed to attention to variability. Doesn't taking *any* drug encourage us to be more aware of our bodies? If so, it is interesting to think about how much of the effectiveness of drugs in general is a result of this attention we pay to our bodies. Perhaps we'll learn that most drugs are not as necessary as we have thought.

The Power of Mindfulness

The research that I've described here (and in my three previous books on mindfulness) makes clear that actively noticing new things is literally and figuratively enlivening. Not only is it not tiring, it is exhilarating. It is the way we feel when we are fully engaged. There seems to me little reason not to begin applying mindfulness to understanding and attempting greater control over our health. There has been new research on the positive effects of meditation that suggest we do so. Psychologist Richard Davidson has been leading the way in showing the changes in our brains that result from meditation and mindfulness.[4]

But mindfulness does not require meditation. Dan Siegal points out in his book *The Mindful Brain* that the contemplative practice of meditation results in no greater health improvements than the more immediate steps to mindfulness that I've studied for over thirty years—attending to variability.[5]

Let's reconsider the idea of viewing our health along multiple criteria instead of seeing ourselves as sick or healthy at any particular time. Rather than accept diagnoses as if disease categories don't overlap—the "you either have it or you don't" approach—

we need to gather information that would help us view ourselves along a continuum. It would make clear that the disease is not all or nothing and remind us that it is more controllable than we might have thought. It is easier to imagine moving along our health continuum than to move from fully sick to fully cured. These multiple continua would convey that we are in some respects always healthy but not invulnerable, so mindful attention to our bodies is more than a part-time job to be entered into only after we become ill. Most important, by showing that on several dimensions there is more of some diseases and less of others, we reinforce the idea that we are not our illness.

If we get at least an idea of where we are on several dimensions and take whatever measures we've used a few more times, we will come to see that these indices don't stand still. Once that happens, we open up the possibility of asking why we are sometimes better, and with that comes the possibility of control.

Not only do we need to actively question the dichotomy of healthy versus sick, but we may prosper from recognizing that health isn't just the absence of illness. Why take where we are when we're not ailing as the best we can be? Who established those upper limits? Many of the studies described in these pages question the limits others take to be wired into our bodies or genetically predetermined. They've questioned whether vision can be improved, whether aging must look the way it currently does, whether exercise has a strong mental component, and whether on many dimensions we can turn the clock back. These studies show us how to fight the negative effects of unconscious primes, question the hidden decisions that rob us of choices, and unpack the way the world has been socially constructed when it doesn't fit us and rebuild it to our own specifications. No one is stopping us from making use of this information.

Whenever we try to heal ourselves and do not abdicate our responsibility completely to doctors, each step is mindful. We welcome new information, whether from our bodies or from books. We look at our illnesses from more than the single perspective of medicine. We work on changing contexts, whether it is a stressful workplace or a depressing view of the hospital. And finally, when we attempt to stay healthy rather than to be made well by the medical world, we become involved in the process rather than just the outcome.

It is this deliberate nature of mindfulness that makes its potential so enormous.

Mindful health is most relevant for the prevention and cure of disease before it becomes serious. At the point of dealing with major depression, a cancer that has already found its way to the major organs of our body, or even an extreme case of ADHD, it is helpful, but the solutions are not as easy. Still, even in these extreme cases, increasing mindfulness can only help. The goal, rather than to feel as we once had when we were younger and fully vital, would be to engage in mindful living until we have taken our last breath. It is a goal worth striving toward and one within our reach—to live all the moments of our lives fully conscious.

The Psychopathologizing of Everyday Life

Instead of mindfully attending to our health, we are a culture bent on the psychopathologizing of everyday life. Instead of recognizing that in certain circumstances sadness is rational, we call ourselves depressed. Rather than recognize that there is more than one view of any situation, we deem people—even ourselves—to be "in denial" if they disagree with the dominant view. If we have a positive view of events, we are told we are rationalizing. Almost every pain becomes a syndrome. How many of us declare that we suffer from insomnia after just one night of little sleep?

Let's explore that last case as an illustration of the rest. For many people, the quiet that comes as soon as we get into bed is actually the best time to problem-solve. The catch is that not all problems are so easily solved. If a solution doesn't come readily and we keep at it, we may be up a good portion of the night. The next day a television commercial might suggest that if we can't sleep, we might not only be suffering from insomnia but also obsessing, and we need to take whatever pill they are selling.

It may be common for people who have to get up very early the next day to go to bed early the night before. If they can't fall asleep right away, it's not because they are suffering from insomnia. The sleep we need is a function of the day we've just experienced and the amount of sleep we got the night before—not some notion of the sleep we'll need in the future. How was it determined that we need eight hours of sleep? Who were the subjects in these studies and what hidden decisions were made in the tests? If so many people are declaring that they can't sleep, perhaps the problem is our expectation about the amount of sleep we need. Shouldn't the amount of sleep necessary depend on how much exercise we got that day before we got into bed and what we ate and experienced, rather than the expectations we put on ourselves?

The disorders we create for ourselves do much to explain our nearly pathological relationship with doctors and the world of medicine. Most people agree that being in the hospital is a stressful experience. To some extent, this belief comes from the fact that physicians are trained to be concerned but detached.

While most physicians surely care about their patients, in a study of medical training, psychologists Harold Lief and Renée Fox found that there was more focus on detachment than concern because dealing with death is so difficult.[6] Yet for most of us, personal relationships go a long way toward reducing our stress and helping us heal. Physicians are taught to be detached so they can carry out difficult procedures that would be harder if they had a meaningful relationship with the patient. Detachment may hide uncertainty. If I cared deeply for you and knew *for sure* that cutting off your arm would save your life (a difficult procedure to carry out, to be sure), I believe I wouldn't hesitate to cut. But since I care so much for you I don't want to be mistaken, and so because of my uncertainty I can't easily follow the prescribed procedure. If detachment helps physicians proceed when they are not sure, do we want them to proceed? Regardless of the answer, relationships are healing and we don't need to accept their detachment. Mindfully engaging physicians will increase the chances that they will respond in kind.

Previously I argued that medical data, while useful, cannot be fully trusted. It should guide rather than govern what we do. We also saw that we cannot trust past experience as though it informs us independent of any perspective. Whether we accept it or not, experience only teaches us what we've already learned to learn. How then should we proceed as health learners? We need to take cues from normative medical data and our own personal past experience and integrate them into our current experience. When we do this mindfully, what we really learn from experience is the experience of being.

My mother, although an intelligent woman, was not a mindful learner. I well remember the day she called to tell me she had heard on the radio that John Wayne had just died. She had been living with breast cancer for the past six months and, scared, she asked me if she was going to die. I told her that she and John Wayne had very little in common, including the kind of cancer they each had. But, more important, I told her that she ought to be the first to know how she feels, not the last. What have we come to as a society that we rely on experts and technology to such an extent that we pay such little heed to the personal information we each have about ourselves, information that others can only guess? While being a mindful health learner might or might not have extended my mother's life, it would have enriched her time while alive.

The Journey to Possibility

This book attempts to describe a journey we each can choose to make, how we have come so far from where we might better be, and how we may return home safely and mindfully. It is a place where we gather and respect personal information to which only we are privy and then use medical information as a guide, rather than absolute truth.

What would happen if we considered all illness to be psychosomatic, as I suggested in the beginning of this book? Would we learn anything new about ourselves and our diseases? Would we be more likely to notice the times we are disease- or symptom-free?

Until a few weeks ago, my father was strong and essentially of sound mind. After a minor heart attack, too many medical procedures, and lots of medication, he became much weaker and confused. The medical world deemed him to be incompetent. If his disorientation was from the drugs he was given, was there anything he could he do that would change people's understanding of his competence? Once an elderly adult is diagnosed, it serves as a lens through which to view who they are. Much of our behavior, no matter how old we are, is idiosyncratic and looks even stranger when viewed through that lens. The research on dementia focuses on the period of time the patient spends disoriented. What would happen if we spent as much time looking at this person when he is functioning perfectly well? We might think to take an MRI when the patient is showing symptoms and compare it with another when he was not showing symptoms. Starting with a view of health rather than sickness leads to a different information search. My father was at that time improving and his faculties had returned. He and I both noticeed it. The diagnosis didn't change, though. Like medical theories, indeed all theories, diagnoses rarely do. In my father's case, all they said was that the progress of the dementia had slowed.

Everything we find today that was presumed to be impossible yesterday could lead to a healthier respect for uncertainty and the general questioning of limits. All too often, however, the new finding only leads to a specific change in the theory generating it. It could do more by questioning the whole idea of limits.

Questioning presumed limits is the essence of the psychology of possibility. Asking why we can't become better even when we feel we are at our best and our healthiest is the only way we will ever know how good we can be. The psychology of possibility takes our desired ends as its starting point. It's not just a matter of asking if we can reverse paralysis, blindness, brain damage, or "terminal" cancer, or even regenerate limbs that we've lost, because we've been taught that we cannot. And as such, the past determines our present. Everything is the same, however, until it is not. When we acknowledge that things change and that once again our current "facts" are not immutable, possibility presents itself. If instead of asking whether we can effectively change any of these we ask how we can do it, we can begin finding out.

The very first step may be to put the mind and body back together again. When they are seen as separate, the importance of the body is often placed above the importance of the mind. And so we drink first to our health and then to our happiness. But as we've seen, our attitudes, ideas, and beliefs are at least as important to health as our diets and our doctors. Our minds are not separate from our bodies. While we object strenuously to people trying to control our minds, we too easily give up control of our bodies. It is time to take back control, to become mindful—to notice subtle changes in our bodies, in our circumstances, and in our relationships, and to help those we care about do the same.

At ninety years of age, my friend Dodi Powell understood the importance of mindfulness to our health and well-being. She knew the benefits that accrue to both when we take charge of our own care. Our last visit, shortly before her death, was particularly important to me because of my abiding interest in old age and my father's life as an elderly adult.

The table beside Dodi's bed held books, a vase of flowers, a mug of pens, medicine, Kleenex, and our cooling cups of tea. We talked about the way many older adults live out their last years. She said comforting words about old age, but she was clearly thinking about the long span of her life. Before we parted she said, "I'm not afraid of dying, Ellen, but living sure can be fun."

We could all be so wise.

ACKNOWLEDGMENTS

On behalf of the reader, I want to thank David Miller—my agent, editor, and dear friend. I have gained enormously from his sharp mind and attention to detail. I'm also grateful to my editor at Ballantine, Marnie Cochran, whose thoughtful questions and helpful suggestions improved the logic of my arguments and made the book an easier read. I would also like to thank my close friends Pamela Painter and Merloyd Lawrence for their invaluable revisions to an earlier draft of this manuscript.

This book is based on research conducted over many years. Not surprisingly, then, there are many past and present students from my lab to whom I am grateful: Benzion Chanowitz, Sarit Golub, Becca Levy, Tal Ben-Shachar, Adam Grant, Laura Delizonna, Allan Filipowicz, Stephan Jacobs, Mark Palmarino, Philip Thayer, Mark Rhodes, Ali Crum, Arin Madenci, Laura Hsu, Jaewoo Chung, Michael Pirson, Rory Gawler, Meghan Pasriche, Long Ouyang, Jim Ritchie-Dunham, Paul Teplitz, Elizabeth Ward, Jane Juliano, and Ryan Williams. They have all enriched the ideas described as well as my intellectual life. I am also grateful to Juliette McClendon for her careful technical assistance.

No one knows from where our ideas come. A supportive academic environment is surely part of the answer. Anthony Greenwald, Richard Hackman, Mahzarin Banaji, Elizabeth Spelke, Susan Carey, Stephen Kosslyn, and Steven Pinker are particularly appreciated in this regard.

Early one evening a few years ago, I received a call from Grant Scharbo about making a movie based on the counterclockwise study described in this book. He went on in an excited way to tell me why I should let him rather than anyone else make a movie based on my life and work. He was charming and persuasive and I was thrilled to hear his plans. He didn't seem to know that there was not a long line ahead of him, but I would have agreed regardless. Because of the movie, the retreat study became the theme around which this book was organized. It is only fitting, then, to express my gratitude to the producers, Grant Scharbo, Gina Mathews, Kristen Hahn, and Jennifer Aniston, and to screenwriter Paul Bernbaum for making this happen.

I'm not one to typically follow convention, but do so now in saving the most important for last. All of my thoughts and life continue to be enriched by Nancy Hemenway. I thank you for your wisdom, kindness, and generosity. Thank you for being.

RECOMMENDED READING

Dan Ariely, *Predictably Irrational: The Hidden Forces That Shape Our Decisions*, New York: HarperCollins, 2008.

Mahzarin Banaji and Anthony Greenwald, *Ordinary Prejudice*, New York: Bantam Dell, 2009.

Tal Ben-Shahar, *Happier: Learn the Secrets to Daily Joy and Lasting Fulfillment*, New York: McGraw-Hill, 2007.

Harold J. Bursztajn, Richard I. Feinbloom, Robert M. Hamm, and Archie Brodsky, *Medical Choices, Medical Chances: How Patients, Families, and Physicians Can Cope With Uncertainty*, New York: Routledge, 1991.

Mihaly Csikszentmihalyi, *Flow: The Psychology of Optimal Experience*, New York: Harper Perennial, 1991.

Atul Gawande, *Complications: A Surgeon's Notes on an Imperfect Science*, New York: Picador, 2003.

Daniel Gilbert, *Stumbling on Happiness*, New York: Vintage Books, 2007.

Ellen J. Langer, *On Becoming an Artist: Reinventing Yourself Through Mindful Creativity*, New York: Ballantine, 2006.

———, *Mindfulness*, Boston: Da Capo Press, 1990.

———, *The Power of Mindful Learning*, Boston: Da Capo Press, 1998.

Steve Pinker, *The Stuff of Thought: Language as a Window into Human Nature*, New York: Viking, 2007.

Martin Seligman, *Authentic Happiness: Using the New Positive Psychology to Realize Your Potential for Lasting Fulfillment*, New York: Free Press, 2004.

Daniel J. Siegal, *The Mindful Brain: Reflection and Attunement in the Cultivation of Well-Being*, New York: W. W. Norton & Company, 2007.

Daniel M. Wegner, *The Illusion of Conscious Will*, Cambridge, MA: MIT Press, 2002.

NOTES

Chapter 1: Counterclockwise

1. E. Langer and J. Rodin, "The effects of enhanced personal responsibility for the aged: a field experiment in an institutional setting," *Journal of Personality and Social Psychology* 34 (1976), pp. 191–98.

2. C. Alexander and E. Langer (eds.), *Higher Stages of Human Development: Perspectives on Adult Growth*, New York: Oxford University Press, 1990. See also C. Alexander, E. Langer, R. Newman, H. Chandler, and J. Davies, "Aging, mindfulness and meditation," *Journal of Personality and Social Psychology* 57 (1989), pp. 950–64.

Chapter 2: Health, Unlimited

1. Leo Tolstoy, *The Death of Ivan Ilych*, New York: Signet Classics, 2004.

2. Eve Weiss, "Dr. Groopman's Prescription: Expert advice on how to diagnose your doctor before he diagnoses you," *02138*, May/June 2007.

3. William James, *The Principles of Psychology*, Cambridge, MA: Harvard University Press, 1983.

4. Bernice Neugarten, "Adult personality: toward a psychology of the life cycle," in Bernice Neugarten (ed.), *Middle Age and Aging*, Chicago: University of Chicago Press, pp. 137–47.

5. David P. Phillips, Camilla A. Van Voorhees, and Todd E. Ruth, "The birthday: lifeline or deadline?" *Psychosomatic Medicine* 54, 5 (1992), pp. 532–42.

6. Sandra Blakeslee, "Birthdays: a matter of life and death," *New York Times*, September 22, 1992.

7. B. R. Levy, M. D. Slade, S. V. Kasl, and S. R. Kunkel, "Longevity increased by positive self-perception of aging," *Journal of Personality and Social Psychology* 83, 2 (2002), pp. 261–70.

8. H. Maier and J. Smith, "Psychological predictors of mortality in old

age," *Journals of Gerontology Series B: Psychological Sciences and Social Sciences* 54B, 1 (1999), pp. 44–54.

9. E. Langer, A. Blank, and B. Chanowitz, "The mindlessness of ostensibly thoughtful action: the role of placebic information in interpersonal interaction," *Journal of Personality and Social Psychology* 36 (1978), pp. 635–42.

10. E. Langer and A. Benevento, "Self-induced dependence," *Journal of Personality and Social Psychology* 36 (1978), pp. 886–93.

Chapter 3: Variability

1. N. E. Miller, "Analytical studies of drive and reward," *American Psychologist* 16 (1961), pp. 739–54.

2. L. Delizonna, R. Williams, and E. Langer, "The effect of mindfulness on heart rate control," *Journal of Adult Development and Aging*, in press.

3. Silvan Tompkins, as quoted by Robert Abelson in personal conversation.

4. L. Burpee and E. Langer, "Mindfulness and marital satisfaction," *Journal of Adult Development* 12 (2005), pp. 43–51.

5. E. Langer, J. Rodin, P. Beck, C. Weinman, and L. Spitzer, "Environmental determinants of memory improvement in late adulthood," *Journal of Personality and Social Psychology* 37 (1979), pp. 2003–13.

6. D. E. Nee, M. G. Berman, K. S. Moore, and J. Jonides, "Neuroscientific evidence on the distinction between short- and long-term memory," *Current Directions in Psychological Science* 17, 2 (2008), p. 102.

Chapter 4: The Social Construction of Health

1. B. Levy and E. Langer, "Shifting the balance of power from nursing home staff to residents," *Nursing Home Economics* (1995).

2. R. L. Atkinson, N. V. Dhurandhar, D. B. Allison, R. L. Bowen, B. A. Israel, J. B. Albu, and A. S. Augustus, "Human adenovirus-36 is associated with increased body weight and paradoxical reduction of serum lipids," *International Journal of Obesity* 29, 3 (2005), pp. 281–86.

3. D. H. Brendel, *Healing and Psychiatry: Bridging the Science/Humanism Divide*, Cambridge, MA: MIT Press, 2006.

4. Ashley Pettus, "Psychiatry by prescription: do psychotropic drugs blur

the boundaries between illness and health?" *Harvard Magazine* 108, 6 (July–August 2006).

5. S. Port, L. Demer, R. Jennrich, D. Walter, and A. Garfinkel, "Systolic blood pressure and mortality," *Lancet* 355, 9199 (2000), pp. 175–80.

6. Robin Marantz Henig, "Fat factors," *New York Times Sunday Magazine*, August 13, 2006.

7. Dorota Gertig, John Hopper, and Graham Giles, "A prospective cohort study of the relationship between physical activity, body size and composition, and the risk of ovarian cancer [Melbourne Collaborative Cohort Study]", *Cancer Epidemiology Biomarkers and Prevention* 13 (2004), pp. 2117–25. See also "Accurate prediction of fracture risk in osteoporotic women," *Medical News Today*, September 28, 2006.

8. K. M. Flegal, B. I. Graubard, D. F. Williamson, and M. H. Gail, "Excess deaths associated with underweight, overweight, and obesity," *Journal of the American Medical Association*, 293 (2005), pp. 1861–67.

9. M. E. P. Seligman and W. R. Miller, "Depression and learned helplessness in man," *Journal of Abnormal Psychology* 84, 3 (1975), pp. 228–38. See also M. E. P. Seligman and S. F. Maier, "Learned helplessness: theory and evidence," *Journal of Experimental Psychology* 105, 1 (1976), pp. 3–46.

10. C. P. Richter, "On the phenomenon of sudden death in animals and man," *Psychosomatic Medicine* 19 (1957), pp. 191–98.

11. C. Peterson, M. E. P. Seligman, and G. E. Vaillant, "Pessimistic explanatory style as a risk factor for physical illness: a thirty-five year longitudinal study," *Journal of Personality and Social Psychology* 55 (1988), pp. 23–27.

12. D. P. Philips, T. E. Ruth, and L. M. Wagner, "Psychology and survival," *Lancet* 342 (1993), pp. 1142–45.

13. S. Cohen, W. J. Doyle, R. B. Turner, C. M. Alper, and D. P. Skoner, "Emotional style and susceptibility to the common cold," *Psychosomatic Medicine* 65, 4 (2003), pp. 652–57.

14. M. Mather, T. Canli, T. English, S. Whitfield, P. Wais, K. Ochsner, J. D. Gabrieli, and L. L. Carstensen, "Amygdala responses to emotionally valenced stimuli in older and younger adults," *Psychological Science* 15, 4 (2004), pp. 259–63.

15. M. F. Scheier and C. S. Carver, "Effects of optimism on psychological and physical well-being: theoretical overview and empirical update," *Cognitive Therapy and Research* 16, 2 (1992), pp. 201–28. See also M. F.

Scheier, K. A. Matthews, and J. F. Owens, "Dispositional optimism and recovery from coronary artery bypass surgery: the beneficial effects on physical and psychological well-being," *Journal of Personality and Social Psychology* 57, 6 (1989), pp. 1024–40.

16. Gerd Gigerenzer, *Calculated Risks*, New York: Simon and Schuster, 2002.

17. R. Tamimi, S. Hankinson, W. Chen, B. Rosner, and G. Colditz, "Combined estrogen and testosterone use and risk of breast cancer in postmenopausal women," *Archives of Internal Medicine* 166 (2006), pp. 1483–89.

18. Sarit Golub, "Optimism, Pessimism, and HIV Risk-Behavior: Motivation or Rationalization?" Harvard University, Department of Psychology, Ph.D. dissertation, 2004.

19. If we were told we didn't have cancer, but were on the borderline, then there would still be a group on the border of our borderline group.

Chapter 5: Reengineering Medical Rules

1. A. G. Greenwald, M. R. Banaji, and L. A. Rudman, "A unified theory of implicit attitudes, stereotypes, self-esteem, and self-concept," *Psychological Review* 109, 1 (2002), pp. 3–25.

2. J. A. Bargh, M. Chen, and L. Burrows, "Automaticity of social behavior: direct effects of trait construct and stereotype activation on action," *Journal of Personality and Social Psychology* 71, 2 (1996), pp. 230–44.

3. M. Djikic, E. J. Langer, and S. F. Stapleton, "Reducing stereotyping through mindfulness: decreasing effects of stereotype-activated behaviors," *Journal of Adult Development* 15 (2008), pp. 106–111.

4. J. Avorn and E. J. Langer, "Induced disability in nursing home patients: a controlled trial," *Journal of the American Geriatrics Society*, 30, 6 (1982), pp. 397–400.

5. E. J. Langer, S. Fiske, and S. E. Taylor, "Stigma, staring, and discomfort: a novel-stimulus hypothesis," *Journal of Experimental Social Psychology* 12, 5 (1976), pp. 451–63.

6. J. Burgoon and E. Langer, "Interpersonal mindlessness and language," *Communication Monographs* 59 (1992), pp. 324–327.

7. E. J. Langer and A. M. Grant, "Putting people back in the equation: the person salience effect," Harvard University, Department of Psychology, 2004.

Chapter 6: Words in Context

1. E. J. Langer and J. Rodin, "The effects of choice and enhanced personal responsibility for the aged: a field experiment in an institutional setting," *Journal of Personality and Social Psychology* 34, 2 (1976), pp. 191–98.

2. J. Bonnefon and G. Villejoubert, "Tactful or doubtful? expectations of politeness explain the severity bias in the interpretation of probability phrases," *Psychological Science* 17, 9 (2006), pp. 747–51.

3. Margaret Shih, Todd Pittinsky, and Nalini Ambady, "Stereotype susceptibility: identity salience and shifts in quantitative performance," *Psychological Science* 10 (1999), pp. 80–83. See also Nalini Ambady, Margaret Shih, Amy Kim, and Todd L. Pittinsky, "Stereotype susceptibility in children: effects of identity activation on quantitative performance," *Psychological Science* 12, 5, (2001), pp. 385–390.

4. B. Levy, "Improving memory in old age through implicit self-stereotyping," *Journal of Personality and Social Psychology* 71, 6 (1996), pp. 1092–107.

5. B. R. Levy, J. M. Hausdorff, R. Hencke, and J. Y. Wei, "Reducing cardiovascular stress with positive self-stereotypes of aging," *Journal of Gerontology Series B: Psychological Sciences and Social Sciences* 55, 4 (2000), pp. 205–13.

6. A. Roefs, C. P. Herman, and C. M. MacLeod, "At first sight: how do restrained eaters evaluate high-fat palatable foods?" *Appetite* 44, 1 (2005), pp. 103–14.

7. B. Shiv, Z. Carmon, and D. Ariely, "Placebo effects of marketing actions: consumers may get what they pay for," *Journal of Marketing Research* 42, 4 (2005), pp. 383–93.

8. Rebecca Waber, Baba Shiv, Ziv Carmon, and Dan Ariely, "Commercial features of placebo and therapeutic efficacy," *Journal of the American Medical Association* 299, 9 (2008); Baba Shiv, Ziv Carmon, and Dan Ariely, "Placebo effects of marketing actions: consumers may get what they pay for," *Journal of Marketing Research* 42, 4 (2005), pp. 383–93.

9. H. M. Lefcourt (ed.), *Locus of Control: Current Trends in Theory and Research*, Hillsdale, NJ: Lawrence Erlbaum Associates, 1982.

10. E. J. Langer, M. Dillon, R. Kurtz, and M. Katz, "Believing Is Seeing," Harvard University, Department of Psychology, 1988.

11. E. J. Langer, M. Djikic, A. Madenci, M. Pirson, and R. Donahue, "Believing is seeing: reversing vision inhibiting mindsets," Harvard University, Department of Psychology, 2009.

12. C. Shawn Green and Daphne Bavelier, "Action video game modifies visual selective attention," *Nature* 423 (2003), pp. 534–37.

13. H. Benson and D. P. McCallie, "Angina pectoris and the placebo effect," *New England Journal of Medicine* 300, 25 (1979), pp. 1424–29.

14. A. H. Roberts, D. G. Kewman, M. Hovell, and L. Mercier, "The power of nonspecific effects in healing: implications for psychosocial and biological treatments," *Clinical Psychology Review* 13, 5 (1993), pp. 375–91.

15. I. Kirsh and G. Sapirstein, "Listening to Prozac but hearing placebo: a meta-analysis of antidepressant medication," *Prevention and Treatment* 1, 2 (1998).

16. S. Blakeslee, "Placebos prove so powerful even experts are surprised," *New York Times*, October 13, 1998. See also K. Nesbitt Shanor, *The Emerging Mind: New Research into the Meaning of Consciousness*, Los Angeles: Renaissance Books, 1999.

17. A. J. Crum and E. J. Langer, "Mind-set matters: exercise and the placebo effect," *Psychological Science* 18, 2 (2007), pp. 165–71.

18. J. N. Morris, J. A. Heady, P. A. Raffle, C. G. Roberts, and J. W. Parks, "Coronary heart-disease and physical activity of work," *Lancet* 265, 6795 (1953), pp. 1053–57.

19. Y. J. Cheng, M. S. Lauer, C. P. Earnest, T. S. Church, J. B. Kampert, L. W. Gibbons, and S. N. Blair, "Heart rate recovery following maximal exercise testing as a predictor of cardiovascular disease and all-cause mortality in men with diabetes," *Diabetes Care* 26, 7 (2003), pp. 2052–57.

20. I. M. Lee, J. E. Manson, C. H. Hennekens, and R. S. Paffenbarger Jr., "Body weight and mortality: a 27-year follow-up of middle-aged men," *Journal of the American Medical Association* 270, 23 (1993), pp. 2823–28.

21. P. Schnorr, H. Scharling, and J. S. Jensen, "Changes in leisure-time physical activity and risk of death: an observational study of 7,000 men and women," *American Journal of Epidemiology* 158, 7 (2003), pp. 639–44.

22. "Physical activity and public health—a recommendation from the Centers for Disease Control and Prevention and the American College of Sports Medicine," *Journal of the American Medical Association*, 273 (1995), pp. 402–7.

23. Deena Skolnick Weisberg, Frank C. Keil, Joshua Goodstein, Elizabeth Rawson, and Jeremy R. Gray, "The seductive allure of neuroscience explanations," *Journal of Cognitive Neuroscience* 20 (2008), pp. 470–77.

24. Gerald Davison and Stuart Valins, "Maintenance of self-attributed and drug-attributed behavior change," *Journal of Personality and Social Psychology* 11 (1969), pp. 25–33.

25. L. Hsu, J. Chung, and E. J. Langer, "The influence of age perception on health and longevity: an archival analysis," Harvard University, Department of Psychology, 2009.

Chapter 7: What's in a Word?

1. S. Carson, E. J. Langer, and A. Flodr, "Remission vs. cure: the effects of labels on health and well-being," manuscript in submission. See also, E. J. Langer, "Cancer: remission or cure?" *Psychology Today* 33, 4 (2000), pp. 28–29. See also S. Carson and E. J. Langer, "Mindfulness and Self Acceptance," *Journal of Rational-Emotive and Cognitive-Behavioral Therapy*, in press.

2. B. Chanowitz and E. J. Langer, "Premature cognitive commitment," *Journal of Personality and Social Psychology* 41, 6 (1981), pp. 1051–63.

3. R. Abelson and E. J. Langer, "A patient by any other name: clinician group difference in labeling bias," *Journal of Consulting and Clinical Psychology* 42, 1 (1974), pp. 4–9.

4. D. L. Rosenhan, "On being sane in insane places," *Science* 179, 4070 (1973), pp. 250–58.

5. Nalini Ambady, Debi LaPlante, Thai Nguyen, Robert Rosenthal, Nigel Chaumeton, and Wendy Levinson, "Surgeons' tone of voice: a clue to malpractice history," *Surgery* 132, 1 (2002), pp. 5–9.

6. E. J. Langer and D. Heffernan, "Mindful managing: confident but uncertain managers," Harvard University, Department of Psychology, 1988.

Chapter 8: Limiting Experts

1. A. C. Edmondson, "Learning from failure in health care: frequent opportunities, pervasive barriers," *Quality and Safety in Healthcare* 13, suppl. II (2006), pp. 3–9.

2. Irving L. Janis, *Victims of Groupthink*, Boston: Houghton Mifflin Company, 1972.

3. A. C. Edmondson, "Speaking up in the operating room: how team leaders promote learning in interdisciplinary action teams," *Journal of Management Studies* 40, 6 (2003), pp. 1419–52.

4. Linda T. Kohn, Janet M. Corrigan, and Molla S. Donaldson (eds.), *To Err Is Human: Building a Safer Health System*, Washington, DC: Committee on Quality of Health Care in America, Institute of Medicine, National Academy Press, 2000.

5. B. Heden, H. Ohlin, R. Rittner, and L. Edenbrant, "Acute myocardial infarction detected in the 12-lead ECG by artificial neural networks," *Circulation* 96, 6 (1997), pp. 1798–802.

6. D. W. Bates, L. L. Leape, and S. Petrycki, "Incidence and preventability of adverse drug events in hospitalized adults," *Journal of General Internal Medicine* 8, 6 (1993), pp. 289–94.

7. Robert B. Cialdini, *Influence: The Psychology of Persuasion*, New York: Collins, 1998.

8. Denise Grady, "Cancer patients, lost in a maze of uneven care," *New York Times*, July 29, 2007.

9. This thought is reminiscent of the sentiments in Dr. Jay Katz's important book, *The Silent World of Doctor and Patient* (Baltimore, MD: Johns Hopkins University Press, 2002), in which he urged patients to be involved in their health care.

Chapter 9: Mindful Aging

1. J. Rodin and E. J. Langer, "Aging labels: the decline of control and the fall of self-esteem," *Journal of Social Issues* 36 (1980), pp. 12–29.

2. M. E. Kite and B. T. Johnson, "Attitudes toward older and younger adults: a meta-analysis," *Psychology and Aging* 3, 3 (1988), pp. 233–44.

3. E. J. Langer, L. Perlmuter, B. Chanowitz, and R. Rubin, "Two new applications of mindlessness theory: aging and alcoholism," *Journal of Aging Studies* 2 (1988), pp. 289–99.

4. E. Langer, "The illusion of incompetence," in L. Perlmuter and R. Monty (eds.), *Choice and Perceived Control*, New Jersey: Lawrence Erlbaum Associates, 1979.

5. B. R. Levy, J. M. Hausdorff, R. Hencke, and J. Y. Wei, "Reducing cardiovascular stress with positive self-stereotypes of aging," *Journals of Gerontology Series B: Psychological Sciences and Social Sciences* 55B, 4 (2000), pp. 205–13.

6. R. Schultz, "The effects of control and predictability on the physiological and psychological well being of the aged," *Journal of Personality and Social Psychology* 33 (1976), pp. 563–73.

7. C. Alexander, E. J. Langer, R. Newman, H. Chandler, and J. Davies,

"Aging, mindfulness and meditation," *Journal of Personality & Social Psychology* 57 (1989), pp. 950–64.

8. E. J. Langer, P. Beck, R. Janoff-Bulman, and C. Timko, "The relationship between cognitive deprivation and longevity in senile and non-senile elderly populations," *Academic Psychology Bulletin* 6 (1984), pp. 211–26.

9. R. Rosenthal and L. Jacobson, *Pygmalion in the Classroom: Teacher Expectation and Pupils' Intellectual Development*, New York: Irvington Publishers, 1992.

10. Alan J. Christensen, John S. Wiebe, Eric G. Benotsch, and William J. Lawton, "Perceived health competence, health locus of control, and patient adherence in renal dialysis," *Cognitive Therapy and Research* 20, 4 (1996), pp. 411–21; N. J. Woodward and B. S. Wallston, "Age and health care beliefs: self-efficacy as a mediator of low desire for control," *Psychology and Aging* 2 (1987), pp. 3–8.

11. L. C. Perlmuter and A. S. Eads, "Control: cognitive and motivational implications," in J. Lomranz, ed., *Handbook of Aging and Mental Health: An Integrative Approach*. New York: Plenum Press, 1998.

12. E. B. Palmore, "Ageism in Canada and the United States," Duke University Center for the Study of Aging and Human Development, 2002.

13. M. M. Baltes and H. Wahl, "The dependency-support script in institutions: generalizations to community settings," *Psychology and Aging* 7, 3 (1992), pp. 409–18.

Chapter 10: Becoming Health Learners

1. James Pennebaker, *Opening Up: The Healing Power of Emotional Expression*, New York: Guilford Press, 1997.

2. C. Willis, "Dogs trained to sniff out bladder cancer," *British Medical Journal* 329 (2004), p. 712. Dr. Carolyn Willis trained six dogs to sniff out bladder cancer. Each dog was given seven urine samples from one cancer patient and six patients who did not have cancer. By chance the dogs would have been successful only 14 percent of the time. Instead the dogs had a success rate of 41 percent.

3. B. Chanowitz and E. Langer, "Knowing more (or less) than you can show: understanding control through the mindlessness/mindfulness distinction," in M.E.P. Seligman and J. Garber (eds.), *Human Helplessness*, New York: Academic Press, 1980.

4. A. Lutz, J. P. Dunner, and R. J. Davidson, "Meditation and the neuro-

science of consciousness: an introduction," in P. Zelizo, M. Moscovitch, and E. Thompson (eds.), *Cambridge Handbook of Consciousness*, New York: Cambridge University Press, 2007. See also Richard J. Davidson and Antoine Lutz, "Buddha's brain: neuroplasticity and meditation," *IEEE Signal Processing Magazine* 176 (2007), pp. 176, 172–74, and Antoine Lutz, Heleen A. Slagter, John D. Dunne, and Richard J. Davidson, "Cognitive-emotional interactions: attention regulation and monitoring in meditation," *Trends in Cognitive Sciences* 12, 4 (2008), pp. 163–69.

5. Dan Siegel, *The Mindful Brain*, New York: W. W. Norton and Company, 2007.

6. H. I. Lief and R. C. Fox, "Training for detached 'concern' in medical students," in H. I. Lief, V. F. Lief, and N. R. Lief (eds.), *The Psychological Basis of Medical Practice*, New York: Harper and Row, 1963.

INDEX

ABOUT THE AUTHOR

ELLEN J. LANGER is the author of more than two hundred research articles and eleven books, including the international bestseller *Mindfulness,* which has been translated into fifteen languages. Among other awards and honors, Dr. Langer is the recipient of a Guggenheim Fellowship, the Award for Distinguished Contributions to Psychology in the Public Interest from the American Psychological Association, the Award for Distinguished Contributions of Basic Science to the Application of Psychology from the American Association of Applied and Preventive Psychology, and the Adult Development and Aging Distinguished Research Achievement Award from the American Psychological Association. A member of the psychology department at Harvard University and a painter, she lives in Cambridge, Massachusetts.

ABOUT THE TYPE

This book was set in Granjon, a modern recutting of a typeface produced under the direction of George W. Jones, who based Granjon's design upon the letter forms of Claude Garamond (1480–1561). The name was given to the typeface as a tribute to the typographic designer Robert Granjon.